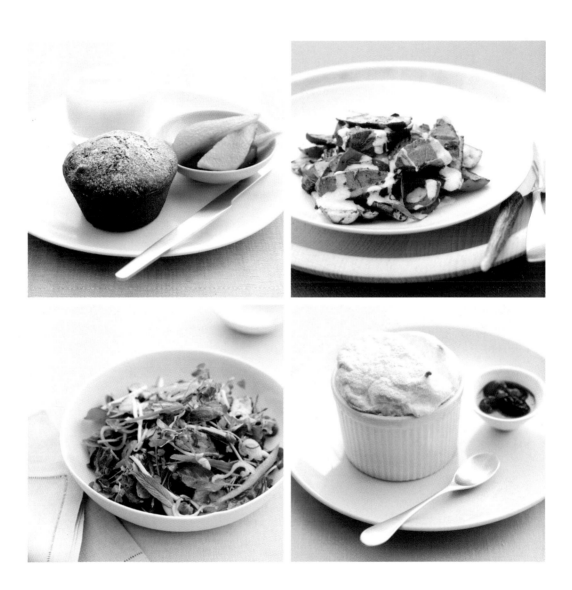

THE AUSTRALIAN

Women's Weekly

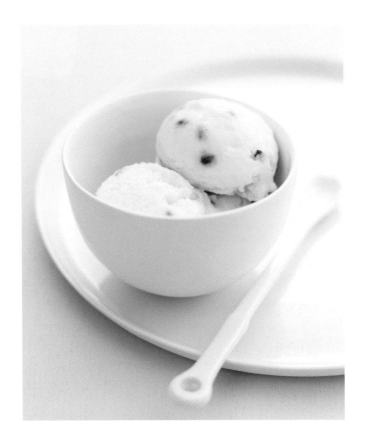

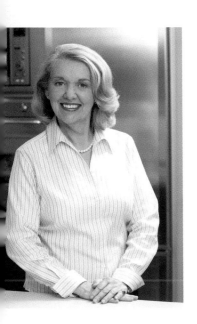

Ever wanted to lose weight? Ever wanted to be slim and trim? Well, look no further – *SLIM* is all you need to start the journey to a healthier you. We have taken the time to cover all meals of the day, from yummy breakfasts to lunchbox ideas that you can pack and assemble at work. We have even included desserts and treats, so whenever you have a craving for something sweet or are feeling peckish, you're able to indulge without piling on extra kilos. So with *SLIM,* get ready for a trimmer and healthier new you.

Pamela Clark

Food Director

contents

introduction   4

breakfast & brunch   6

lunches from home   18

mains   26

desserts   90

treats   106

glossary   116

index   118

facts + figures   119

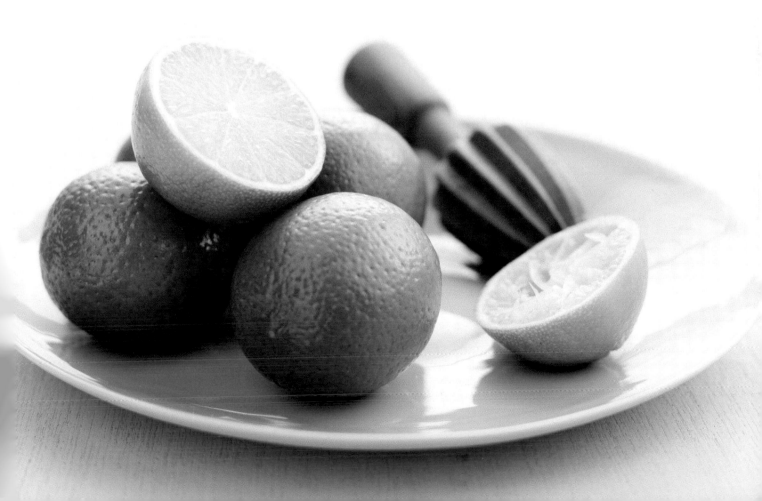

real cooking for a real life

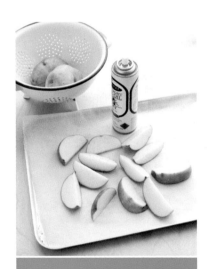

Don't even think about deep-frying. Try, instead, to roast "chips" on a baking-paper-lined oven tray, spraying them with a light coating of olive oil.

Diet is not synonymous with deprivation, despite what a lot of self-help pundits would have you believe. And reducing your fat intake doesn't mean you have to eliminate fats altogether. It's easy to eat well without taking a degree in nutrition; without leaving out the "good stuff" and replacing it with packaged, chemical or artificial substitutes; without spending hours making special dietary dishes no one else in the family will touch; and ... without going without.

Every year "new" nutritional advice changes and contradicts most of the trends and beliefs that have gone before. But there does seem to be one given in the midst of it all, and it's quite simple: eating reasonably sized, well-balanced meals and taking moderate exercise regularly will help keep you happy, healthy and of a constant weight that's right for your age, build and gender.

We all know what happens when we go on a radical diet and the weight just falls away: the minute we go off the diet and back to our normal eating habits, the weight reappears – faster, greater – and we're back on the same relentless treadmill again.

This book aims to put a halt to the feast or famine routine that traps so many of us. Filled with delicious meal ideas that don't baulk at the inclusion of fats or carbs, and recipes providing alternative suggestions to the "bad" content of some of our traditional dishes, *SLIM* isn't a DIET book. It contains no lists of what you can or cannot eat, no daily consumption chart, no incontrovertible rules. What you will find here, however, is real cooking for real life.

One key word to remember in the search for maintaining your healthy weight is "regular". Eat regular meals; don't graze or snack in between. Exercise regularly; a couch-potato lifestyle slows your basic metabolism so you'll

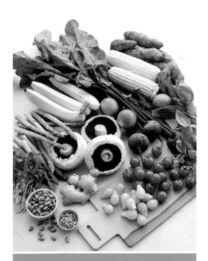

Focus on fibre: eat lots of whole grains, fruit, vegetables and proteins.

need to impose more stringent restrictions on your dietary intake. Your body's energy consumption increases with exercise so, by sticking to a sensible healthy eating plan, you will gradually lose weight – and keep it off – from your early 20s through and beyond your menopausal years.

The breakfast, brunch, dessert and treat recipes in *SLIM* have been developed to contain around 7g of fat per serving; packed lunches are based on around 15g of fat per serving, while main meal recipes can contain up to 20g of fat per serving. This means you can mix and match one selection from each chapter, keeping in mind your daily fat intake should be a maximum of 56g in order to maintain weight.

Consuming more fat per day can lead to an increase in weight, while reducing the amount to about 40g per day, when coupled with exercise, will see the beginning of moderate weight loss.

Try not to eat takeaway food, especially commercial cakes and biscuits, which are among the worst sources of the combination of refined sugar and saturated fats.

Whenever possible, stir-fry in a wok instead of shallow-frying. Heat the wok first before giving the sides a light spray of canola oil.

Try to only ever use olive oil or canola oil for cooking, and use it sparingly.

Stock, water or juice can be used instead of oil or butter to soften some ingredients in soups, sauces and casseroles.

Soups, sauces and casseroles can be thickened with pureed vegetables rather than flour or egg.

Make soups, sauces and casseroles a day ahead, refrigerate them overnight, then skim away the fat that solidifies on the surface before reheating.

Eat smaller portions to help prevent your body from storing excess kilojoules.

Increase your consumption of fish, including canned fish.

Discard the skin from all poultry.

Use low-fat or light dairy products.

Keep only good foods in the house: you won't brave the elements just to go out to buy a tub of chocolate ice-cream.

Keep track of what you eat in a single day by writing everything down in a small notepad that you keep with you.

Drink lots of natural water and get enough sleep.

Don't be impatient: one week's worth of exercise will not turn you into Elle Macpherson. Nothing happens overnight.

BREAKFAST & BRUNCH

Start the day in the best
of ways with fine food
for the body and soul.

soufflé with berry compote

PREPARATION TIME 10 MINUTES   **COOKING TIME** 15 MINUTES   **SERVES** 4

1 tablespoon caster sugar

2 eggs, separated

½ cup (80g) icing sugar mixture

2 egg whites

BERRY COMPOTE

½ cup (75g) frozen mixed berries

2 tablespoons orange juice

1 tablespoon caster sugar

1 Make berry compote.
2 Preheat oven to moderate. Lightly grease four 1¼-cup (310ml) ovenproof dishes; sprinkle insides of dishes evenly with caster sugar, shake away excess. Place dishes on oven tray.
3 Whisk egg yolks and 2 tablespoons of the icing sugar in large bowl until mixture is well combined.
4 Beat the four egg whites in small bowl with electric mixer until soft peaks form. With motor operating, gradually add remaining icing sugar, beating until firm peaks form.
5 Gently fold egg-white mixture, in two batches, into yolk mixture; divide mixture among prepared dishes. Bake soufflés, uncovered, in moderate oven about 12 minutes or until puffed and browned lightly. Dust with sifted icing sugar, if desired; serve with compote.

BERRY COMPOTE Combine ingredients in small saucepan; bring to a boil. Reduce heat; simmer, uncovered, 2 minutes.

NUTRITIONAL INFORMATION PER SERVING

2.7g total fat (0.8g saturated fat) **698kJ (167 cal)** 31.5g carbohydrate **5.4g protein** 0.7g fibre

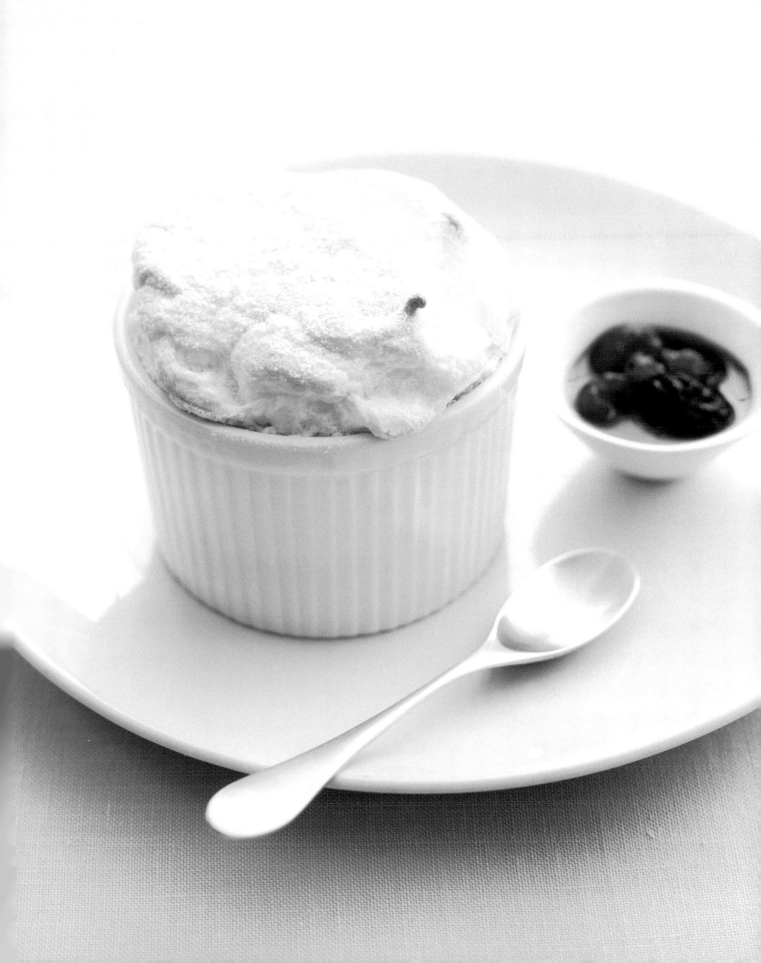

sautéed mushrooms on toast

PREPARATION TIME 10 MINUTES **COOKING TIME** 20 MINUTES **SERVES** 4

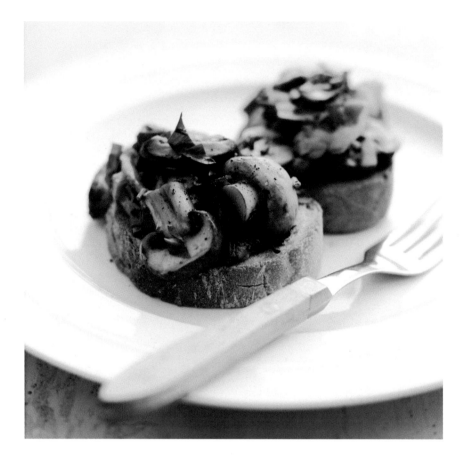

30g butter

200g swiss brown mushrooms, sliced thickly

100g fresh shiitake mushrooms, sliced thickly

200g button mushrooms, halved

100g oyster mushrooms, halved

1 clove garlic, crushed

¼ cup (60ml) beef stock

½ loaf ciabatta (220g)

¼ cup coarsely chopped fresh flat-leaf parsley

¼ cup coarsely chopped fresh chives

1 Preheat grill.

2 Melt butter in large frying pan; cook mushrooms and garlic, stirring, about 5 minutes. Add stock; bring to a boil. Reduce heat; simmer, uncovered, about 10 minutes or until mushrooms are cooked as desired.

3 Meanwhile, trim end from bread; cut into eight slices. Toast bread both sides; divide among serving plates.

4 Stir herbs into mushrooms; serve on toast.

NUTRITIONAL INFORMATION PER SERVING

8.1g total fat (4.3g saturated fat) **966kJ (231 cal)** 29.7g carbohydrate **9.8g protein** 6.2g fibre

poached eggs on sourdough

PREPARATION TIME 5 MINUTES **COOKING TIME** 15 MINUTES **SERVES** 4

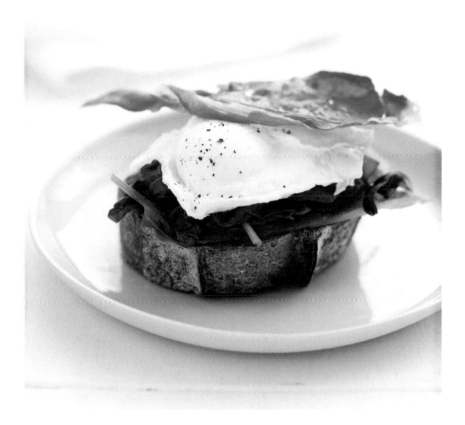

1 Preheat grill.
2 Half-fill large shallow frying pan with water; bring to a boil. Break eggs into cup, one at a time, then slide into pan. When all eggs are in pan, allow water to return to a boil. Cover pan, turn off heat; stand about 4 minutes or until a light film sets over egg yolks. Remove eggs, one at a time, using slotted spoon; place spoon on absorbent-paper-lined saucer briefly to blot up any poaching liquid.
3 Meanwhile, cook prosciutto, in single layer, under preheated grill.
4 Boil, steam or microwave spinach until just wilted; drain. Using hand, squeeze excess water from spinach.
5 Meanwhile, trim end from bread; cut into four slices. Toast bread both sides; divide among serving plates. Top each with 1 slice prosciutto, a quarter of the spinach and an egg, then top with second slice prosciutto.

4 eggs
8 slices prosciutto (120g)
50g baby spinach leaves
½ loaf sourdough (335g)

NUTRITIONAL INFORMATION PER SERVING

9.2g total fat (2.6g saturated fat) **1313kJ (314 cal)** 38g carbohydrate **19.6g protein** 4.2g fibre

oaty apple pikelets

PREPARATION TIME 10 MINUTES (PLUS REFRIGERATION TIME) **COOKING TIME** 15 MINUTES **SERVES** 4

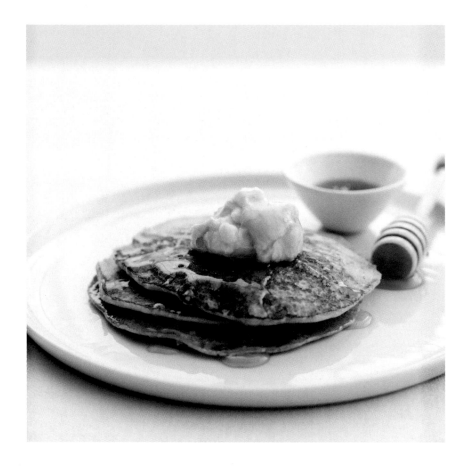

2 cups (500ml) skim milk

1 cup (120g) oat bran

½ cup (75g) plain flour

2 tablespoons brown sugar

½ teaspoon mixed spice

2 eggs

1 large apple (200g), peeled, cored, chopped finely

1 tablespoon lemon juice

½ cup (175g) honey

½ cup (100g) low-fat ricotta

1 Blend or process milk, bran, flour, sugar, spice and eggs until smooth; pour into large jug. Stir in apple and juice, cover; refrigerate 30 minutes (mixture will separate during refrigeration).

2 Heat lightly oiled large frying pan. Stir mixture to combine; using ¼-cup batter for each pikelet (mixture will be runny), cook two pikelets at a time, uncovered, until bubbles appear on the surface. Turn; cook until browned lightly. Remove pikelets from pan; cover to keep warm. Repeat with remaining batter to make 12 pikelets.

3 Divide pikelets among plates; top with honey and ricotta.

NUTRITIONAL INFORMATION PER SERVING

7.3g total fat (2.7g saturated fat) **1973kJ (472 cal)** 83.6g carbohydrate **19g protein** 6.3g fibre

day-before ginger muffins with stewed pear

PREPARATION TIME 25 MINUTES (PLUS REFRIGERATION TIME) **COOKING TIME** 30 MINUTES **MAKES** 6

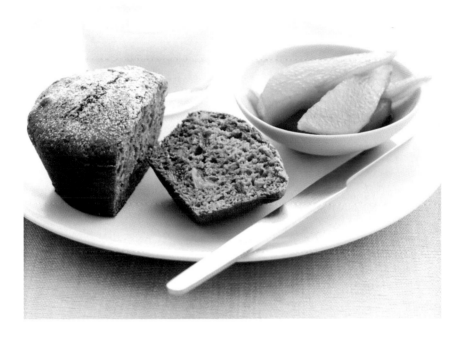

Make the batter for these muffins the night before you want to bake and serve them.

1 Combine ginger, apricot, fig, cereal, milk, brown sugar and half of the golden syrup in large bowl; mix well. Cover; refrigerate overnight.
2 Preheat oven to moderately hot. Lightly grease six-hole (¾-cup/180ml) texas muffin pan.
3 Stir flour and nuts into apricot mixture. Spoon mixture into prepared muffin pan; bake, uncovered, in moderately hot oven about 30 minutes. Stand muffins in pan 5 minutes before turning onto wire rack.
4 Meanwhile, combine pear, remaining golden syrup and the water in large frying pan; simmer, covered, about 15 minutes or until pears are soft. Dust muffins with sifted icing sugar; serve with stewed pear.

3 teaspoons ground ginger

⅔ cup (100g) coarsely chopped dried apricots

½ cup (95g) coarsely chopped dried figs

1⅓ cups (95g) All-Bran breakfast cereal

1½ cups (375ml) skim milk

1¼ cups (275g) firmly packed brown sugar

⅓ cup (115g) golden syrup

1¼ cups (185g) self-raising flour

¼ cup (35g) toasted pecans, chopped coarsely

3 medium pears (690g), peeled, cut into 8 wedges each

1 cup (250ml) water

1 tablespoon icing sugar mixture

NUTRITIONAL INFORMATION PER MUFFIN

5.7g total fat (0.5g saturated fat) **2383kJ (570 cal)** 122.8g carbohydrate **10.1g protein** 12.9g fibre

peach bircher muesli

PREPARATION TIME 25 MINUTES (PLUS REFRIGERATION TIME) **SERVES** 4

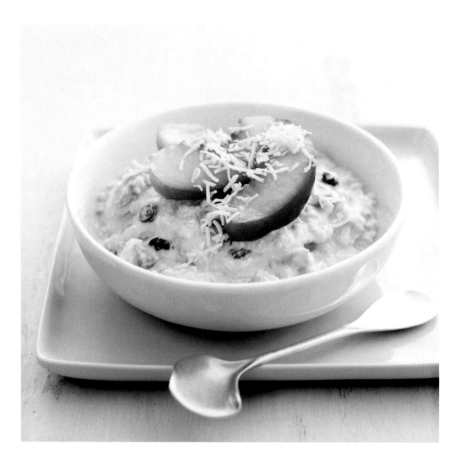

2 cups (220g) natural muesli

1⅓ cups (330ml) apple juice

¾ cup (200g) low-fat country-style yogurt

1¼ cups (185g) dried peaches, chopped coarsely

2 tablespoons honey

¾ cup (180ml) skim milk

1 medium pear (230g), peeled, grated

1 large peach (220g), cut into wedges

¼ cup (15g) toasted shredded coconut

1 Combine muesli, juice, yogurt, dried peach, honey and milk in large bowl. Cover; refrigerate overnight.
2 Stir pear into muesli mixture; serve topped with peach wedges and sprinkled with coconut.

NUTRITIONAL INFORMATION PER SERVING

8.6g total fat (4.2g saturated fat) **2002kJ (479 cal)** 88.1g carbohydrate **13g protein** 12.5g fibre

rice porridge with dried fruit compote

PREPARATION TIME 10 MINUTES (PLUS STANDING TIME) **COOKING TIME** 25 MINUTES **SERVES** 4

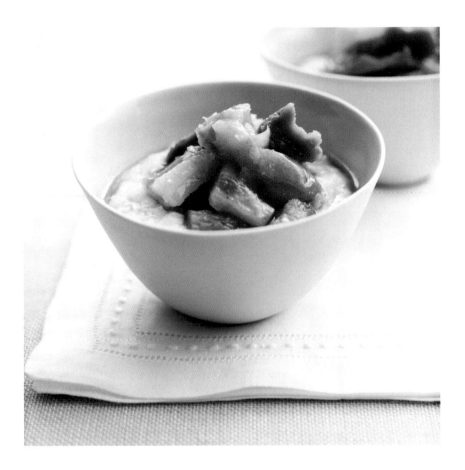

Rolled rice is a gluten-free flaked cereal similar to, and a good substitute for, rolled oats. It is available in supermarkets and health-food stores.

1 Cover rolled rice with the water in small bowl; stand overnight.
2 Make dried fruit compote.
3 Place undrained rolled rice in medium saucepan; cook, stirring, until mixture comes to a boil. Add milk, reduce heat; simmer, uncovered, 10 minutes. Serve with compote.

DRIED FRUIT COMPOTE Halve vanilla bean lengthways, place in medium saucepan with remaining ingredients; bring to a boil. Reduce heat; simmer, uncovered, 20 minutes. Remove from heat; cool 10 minutes. Remove vanilla bean and cinnamon stick before serving.

¾ cup (75g) rolled rice

1½ cups (375ml) water

1 cup (250ml) skim milk

DRIED FRUIT COMPOTE

1 vanilla bean

2½ cups (625ml) water

½ cup (75g) coarsely chopped dried apricots

½ cup (75g) coarsely chopped dried pears

⅓ cup (50g) coarsely chopped dried peaches

2 tablespoons honey

1 teaspoon finely grated lemon rind

1 cinnamon stick

NUTRITIONAL INFORMATION PER SERVING

1.9g total fat (0.4g saturated fat) **1028kJ (246 cal)** 51.5g carbohydrate **6.5g protein** 5.9g fibre

bruschetta with strawberry, banana and ricotta

PREPARATION TIME 15 MINUTES **COOKING TIME** 10 MINUTES **SERVES** 4

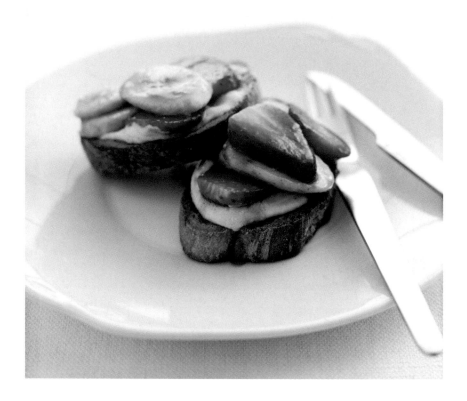

½ **loaf ciabatta (220g)**

200g **low-fat ricotta**

2 **tablespoons honey**

1 **teaspoon finely grated orange rind**

¼ **teaspoon ground cinnamon**

125g **strawberries, sliced thickly**

1 **small banana (130g), sliced thinly**

2 **tablespoons brown sugar**

1 Preheat grill.

2 Trim end from bread; cut into eight slices.

3 Beat ricotta, honey, rind and cinnamon in small bowl with electric mixer until smooth.

4 Combine strawberries, banana and sugar in small frying pan; stir gently over low heat until sugar dissolves.

5 Meanwhile, toast bread both sides. Spread with ricotta mixture, divide among plates; top with strawberry mixture.

NUTRITIONAL INFORMATION PER SERVING

5.8g total fat (3g saturated fat) **1208kJ (289 cal)** 49g carbohydrate **10.8g protein** 2.8g fibre

bruschetta with smoked salmon, cream cheese and rocket

PREPARATION TIME 15 MINUTES **COOKING TIME** 5 MINUTES **SERVES** 4

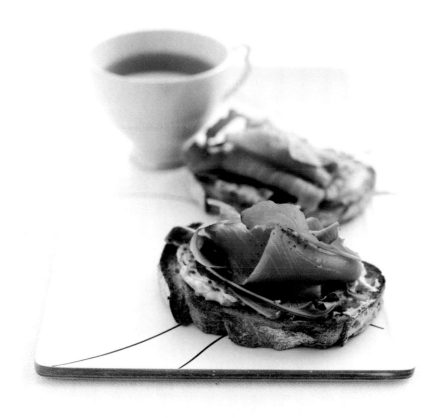

1 Preheat grill.
2 Combine cream cheese, shallot, juice, mustard and capers in small bowl.
3 Trim ends from bread, cut into eight slices. Toast bread both sides. Spread cheese mixture over toast; divide among plates. Top with rocket and salmon.

⅓ cup (80g) light cream cheese

1 shallot (25g), chopped finely

2 teaspoons lemon juice

½ teaspoon dijon mustard

1 tablespoon drained capers, rinsed, chopped coarsely

1 loaf sourdough (675g)

30g baby rocket leaves

200g sliced smoked salmon

NUTRITIONAL INFORMATION PER SERVING

10.1g total fat (3.3g saturated fat) **2153kJ (515 cal)** 77.1g carbohydrate **28g protein** 8g fibre

maple-syrup-flavoured borlotti beans with bacon

PREPARATION TIME 10 MINUTES (PLUS STANDING TIME) **COOKING TIME** 1 HOUR 40 MINUTES **SERVES** 4

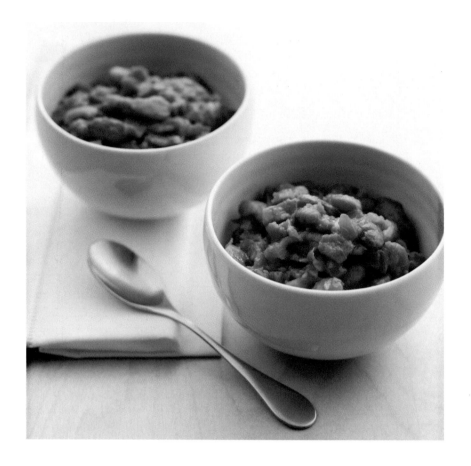

1 cup (200g) dried borlotti beans

3 bacon rashers (210g), rind removed, chopped coarsely

1 medium brown onion (150g), chopped finely

1 clove garlic, crushed

1 tablespoon tomato paste

425g can crushed tomatoes

2 cups (500ml) water

1 tablespoon worcestershire sauce

2 teaspoons dijon mustard

2 tablespoons pure maple syrup

You can soak the beans early in the day before you want to serve them, then at night make this recipe; reheat the beans for breakfast the following day.

1 Place beans in medium bowl, cover with water; stand overnight.
2 Cook bacon, onion and garlic in lightly oiled large saucepan, stirring, until onion softens. Add rinsed, drained beans, paste, undrained tomatoes, the water, sauce and mustard; bring to a boil. Reduce heat; simmer, covered, about 1½ hours or until beans are just tender. Stir maple syrup into hot beans before serving.

NUTRITIONAL INFORMATION PER SERVING

7.6g total fat (2.9g saturated fat) **1032kJ (247 cal)** 30.3g carbohydrate **16.2g protein** 4g fibre

eggs ranchero-style

PREPARATION TIME 10 MINUTES **COOKING TIME** 30 MINUTES **SERVES** 4

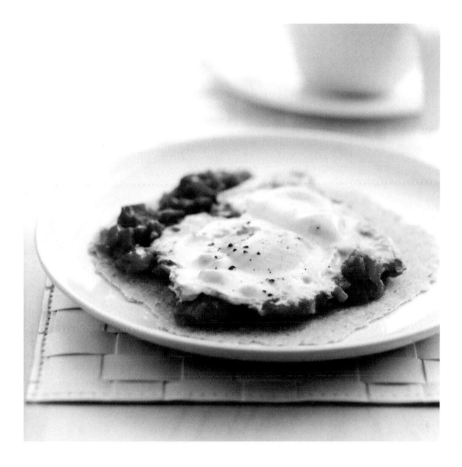

This is our take on the traditional Mexican breakfast dish, huevos rancheros.

1 Cook onion in lightly oiled large non-stick frying pan, stirring, until softened. Add tomato, the water and vinegar; bring to a boil. Reduce heat; simmer, uncovered, 15 minutes, stirring occasionally. Add capsicum; cook, uncovered, 5 minutes.
2 Using large shallow mixing spoon, press four shallow depressions into tomato mixture. Working quickly, break eggs, one at a time, into cup, sliding each egg into one of the hollows in tomato mixture. Cover pan; cook over low heat, about 5 minutes or until eggs are just set.
3 Divide warmed tortillas among plates. Use egg slide to carefully lift egg and tomato mixture onto each tortilla.

1 small red onion (100g), chopped finely

4 medium tomatoes (600g), chopped coarsely

2 tablespoons water

1 tablespoon balsamic vinegar

1 medium red capsicum (200g), chopped finely

4 eggs

4 corn tortillas

NUTRITIONAL INFORMATION PER SERVING

6g total fat (1.7g saturated fat) **619kJ (148 cal)** 13.1g carbohydrate **10.1g protein** 3.4g fibre

LUNCHES FROM HOME

Several of these lunch suggestions help in using up leftovers from the night before. Pack the various components of each recipe in separate containers or snap-lock bags, then mix, dress or heat them, as instructed, at work. Each of the following recipes makes enough for one person.

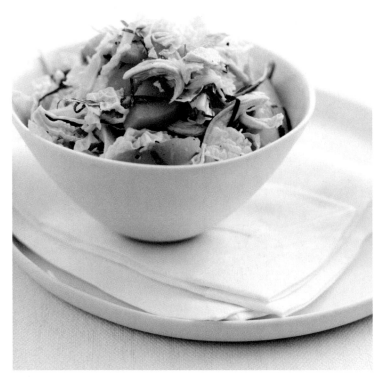

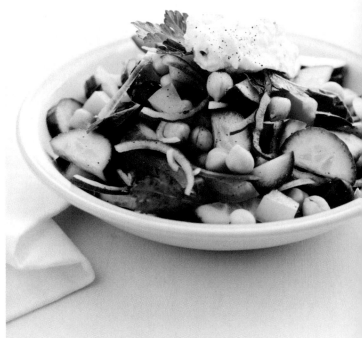

chicken and peach salad

PREPARATION TIME 10 MINUTES

Combine 80g shredded cooked chicken, 1½ cups shredded chinese cabbage, ¼ cup shredded fresh mint leaves and one small peach, cut into wedges. Combine 2 tablespoons lime juice and 1 teaspoon olive oil; toss dressing with salad.

NUTRITIONAL INFORMATION PER SERVING

11.3g total fat (2.4g saturated fat) **974kJ (233 cal)**
8.5g carbohydrate **22.9g protein** 4.4g fibre

chickpea salad

PREPARATION TIME 15 MINUTES

Combine ½ cup rinsed, drained canned chickpeas, one coarsely chopped lebanese cucumber, half a thinly sliced small red onion, ¼ cup seeded kalamata olives, ⅓ cup fresh flat-leaf parsley leaves, ¼ cup coarsely chopped yellow capsicum and one small egg tomato, seeded and cut into wedges. Combine 1 tablespoon lemon juice, 1 teaspoon olive oil, ¼ teaspoon finely chopped lemon rind and ¼ teaspoon ground cumin; toss dressing with salad. Top with 2 tablespoons prepared low-fat tzatziki.

NUTRITIONAL INFORMATION PER SERVING

8.5g total fat (1.6g saturated fat) **1195kJ (286 cal)**
9.8g carbohydrate **11.4g protein** 9g fibre

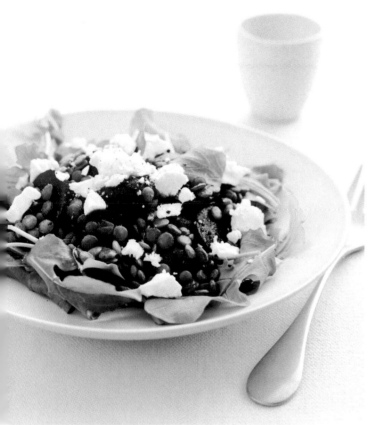

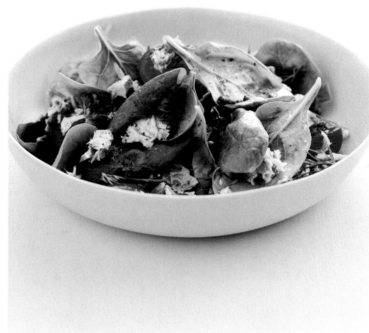

lentil, beetroot and rocket salad

PREPARATION TIME 10 MINUTES

Combine ½ cup cooked brown lentils and ½ cup drained canned baby beetroot halves. Combine 1 tablespoon balsamic vinegar and 1 teaspoon olive oil; toss dressing with salad. Serve on 1½ cups trimmed baby rocket leaves; top with 30g crumbled fetta cheese.

tuna salad

PREPARATION TIME 5 MINUTES

Combine 125g can drained sliced tuna in springwater, 2 cups trimmed baby spinach leaves, 1½ teaspoons rinsed drained baby capers, ⅓ cup halved cherry tomatoes and 3 teaspoons fresh dill sprigs. Combine 1 tablespoon lemon juice and 1 teaspoon olive oil; toss dressing with salad.

NUTRITIONAL INFORMATION PER SERVING

12.6g total fat (5.3g saturated fat) **1041kJ (249 cal)**
19.2g carbohydrate **15.1g protein** 7g fibre

NUTRITIONAL INFORMATION PER SERVING

7.5g total fat (1.7g saturated fat) **798kJ (191 cal)**
3.4g carbohydrate **27.1g protein** 2.8g fibre

19

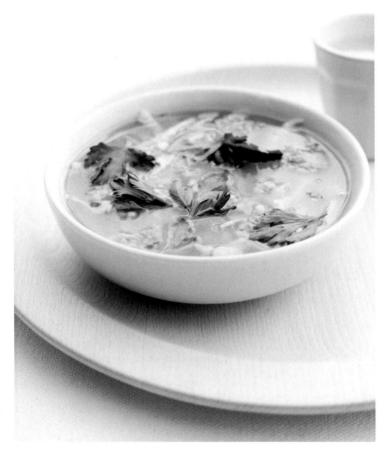

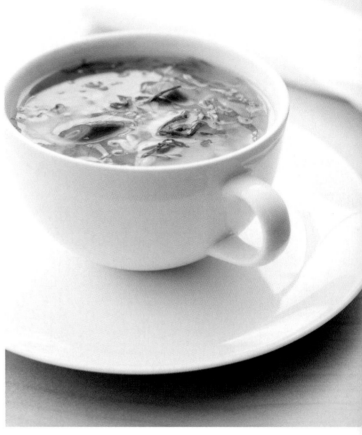

chicken and corn soup

PREPARATION TIME 5 MINUTES
COOKING TIME 2 MINUTES

At home, combine 125g can creamed corn, ½ cup shredded cooked chicken, 1 tablespoon soy sauce and ½ teaspoon sambal oelek. At lunchtime, place corn mixture in medium microwave-safe bowl with 375ml carton salt-reduced chicken stock. Cook, uncovered, on HIGH (100%) in microwave oven about 2 minutes or until hot. Sprinkle with 2 tablespoons fresh flat-leaf parsley leaves.

risoni and spring vegetable soup

PREPARATION TIME 5 MINUTES
COOKING TIME 10 MINUTES

At home, cook ¼ cup risoni in small saucepan of boiling water, uncovered, until almost tender. Add two thinly sliced green beans and one thinly sliced small carrot; cook, uncovered, 1 minute. Drain; rinse under cold water, then drain again. At lunchtime, place risoni mixture in medium microwave-safe bowl with 375ml carton salt-reduced chicken or vegetable stock. Cook, uncovered, on HIGH (100%) in microwave oven about 2 minutes or until hot. Sprinkle with 1 tablespoon shredded fresh basil.

NUTRITIONAL INFORMATION PER SERVING

7.4g total fat (2.4g saturated fat) **1024kJ (245 cal)**
20.4g carbohydrate **24g protein** 4g fibre

NUTRITIONAL INFORMATION PER SERVING

2.2g total fat (0.9g saturated fat) **1016kJ (243 cal)**
44.2g carbohydrate **11g protein** 4.6g fibre

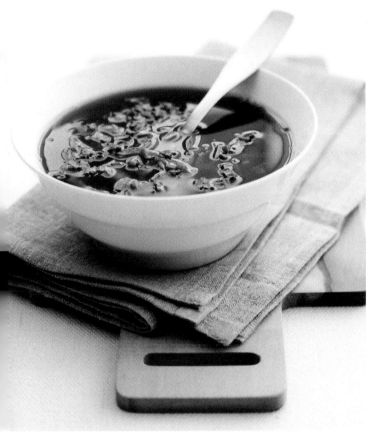

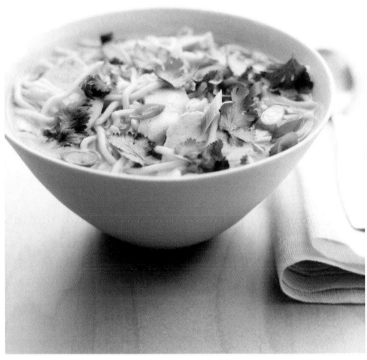

french onion soup

PREPARATION TIME 5 MINUTES
COOKING TIME 15 MINUTES

At home, cook one thinly sliced medium brown onion in 2 teaspoons olive oil in small frying pan, stirring, until onion softens. Add 2 teaspoons brown sugar, then continue to cook, stirring occasionally, about 10 minutes or until onion caramelises. At lunchtime, place onion mixture in medium microwave-safe bowl with 375ml carton salt-reduced beef stock. Cook, uncovered, on HIGH (100%) in microwave oven about 2 minutes or until hot. Sprinkle with 1 teaspoon coarsely chopped fresh chives.

thai chicken noodle soup

PREPARATION TIME 5 MINUTES
COOKING TIME 2 MINUTES

At home, combine ½ cup thinly sliced cooked chicken and 1 teaspoon red curry paste. At lunchtime, rinse 175g packet singapore noodles under hot water. Place noodles in medium microwave-safe bowl with chicken mixture and 375ml carton salt-reduced chicken stock. Cook, uncovered, on HIGH (100%) in microwave oven about 2 minutes or until hot. Sprinkle with 1 tablespoon coarsely chopped fresh coriander and half a thinly sliced green onion.

NUTRITIONAL INFORMATION PER SERVING

10g total fat (1.7g saturated fat) **702kJ (168 cal)**
13.6g carbohydrate **6.5g protein** 1.8g fibre

NUTRITIONAL INFORMATION PER SERVING

10.4g total fat (2.8g saturated fat) **2617kJ (626 cal)**
94g carbohydrate **37.7g protein** 24.4g fibre

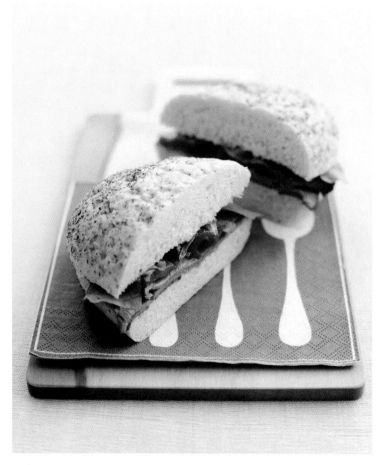

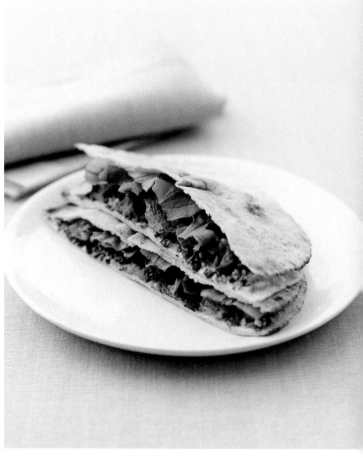

roast beef and horseradish cream on focaccia

PREPARATION TIME 5 MINUTES

Split one small focaccia in half horizontally.
Spread 2 teaspoons horseradish cream on
cut-side of one half of focaccia, then top with
50g sliced roast beef, ¼ cup thickly sliced
char-grilled capsicum, ¼ cup trimmed baby
rocket leaves and remaining half of focaccia.

lamb, tabbouleh and hummus on pitta

PREPARATION TIME 5 MINUTES

Separate one pocket pitta into halves. Spread
1 tablespoon prepared hummus on inside of
one half of pitta, then top with ¼ cup prepared
tabbouleh, 50g sliced roast lamb, ¼ cup trimmed
baby rocket leaves and remaining half of pitta.

NUTRITIONAL INFORMATION PER SERVING

11.4g total fat (2.8g saturated fat) **2165kJ (518 cal)**
72.5g carbohydrate **29.6g protein** 10.6g fibre

NUTRITIONAL INFORMATION PER SERVING

14.6g total fat (4.3g saturated fat) **1772kJ (424 cal)**
48.2g carbohydrate **24.7g protein** 5.9g fibre

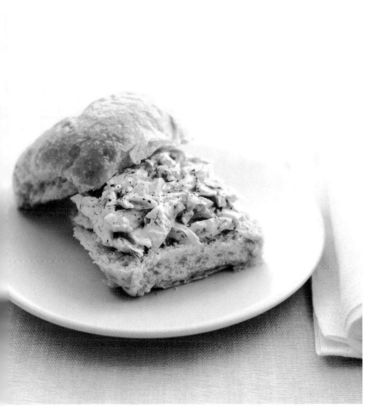

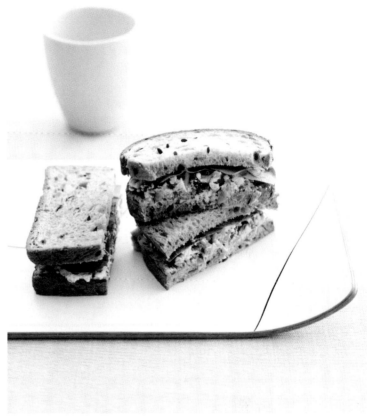

smoked trout salad roll

PREPARATION TIME 5 MINUTES

Split one wholemeal roll in half horizontally. Spread one half with combined 50g flaked smoked trout, 1 tablespoon light sour cream, 1 tablespoon finely chopped cornichons, 1 tablespoon finely chopped fresh dill and 1 tablespoon lemon juice. Top with remaining half of roll.

pea, ricotta, mint and spinach sandwich

PREPARATION TIME 10 MINUTES
COOKING TIME 5 MINUTES

At home, boil, steam or microwave ¼ cup frozen peas until tender; drain. Cool, then, using fork, lightly crush peas. Combine pea mash with 50g low-fat ricotta, 1 tablespoon lemon juice and 1 tablespoon finely chopped fresh mint. At lunchtime, spread pea mixture on one slice soy and linseed bread; top with a few spinach leaves, then sandwich together with another slice soy and linseed bread.

NUTRITIONAL INFORMATION PER SERVING

9.4g total fat (3.7g saturated fat) **1350kJ (323 cal)**
37.5g carbohydrate **21.2g protein** 7g fibre

NUTRITIONAL INFORMATION PER SERVING

9g total fat (3.4g saturated fat) **1195kJ (286 cal)**
33.2g carbohydrate **18.1g protein** 7.9g fibre

Each of these recipes calls for two slices (70g) of ciabatta, a crisp-crusted, soft white Italian bread.

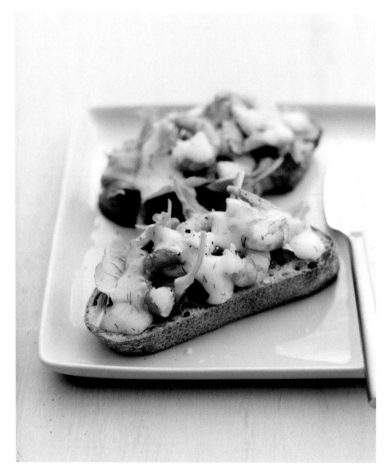

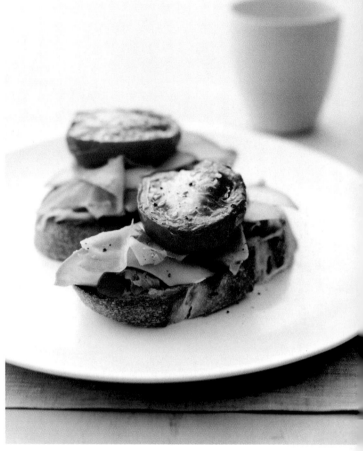

prawn and lime mayonnaise bruschetta

PREPARATION TIME 10 MINUTES
COOKING TIME 2 MINUTES

At home, make lime mayonnaise by combining 2 tablespoons low-fat mayonnaise, 2 teaspoons finely chopped fresh dill and 1 tablespoon lime juice. At lunchtime, toast two slices ciabatta; divide 10g baby rocket leaves, eight cooked small prawns and mayonnaise mixture between both slices.

ham, tomato and avocado bruschetta

PREPARATION TIME 5 MINUTES
COOKING TIME 25 MINUTES

At home, preheat oven to moderate. Place one halved medium egg tomato, cut-side up, on oven tray, sprinkle with 2 teaspoons brown sugar; cook, uncovered, in moderate oven for 20 minutes. At lunchtime, toast two slices ciabatta; divide a quarter of a small avocado, 50g shaved ham and tomato halves between slices. Sprinkle with pepper, if desired.

NUTRITIONAL INFORMATION PER SERVING

7.6g total fat (1.4g saturated fat) **1158kJ (277 cal)**
39.2g carbohydrate **11.9g protein** 2.5g fibre

NUTRITIONAL INFORMATION PER SERVING

11.6g total fat (2.7g saturated fat) **1367kJ (327 cal)**
39.1g carbohydrate **16.6g protein** 3.4g fibre

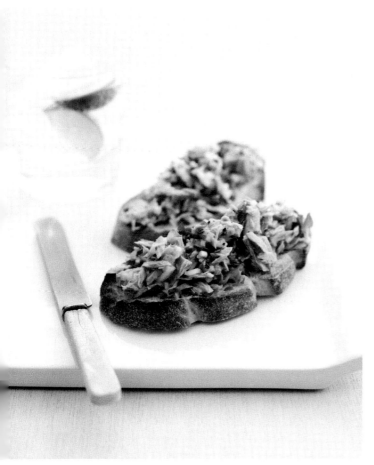

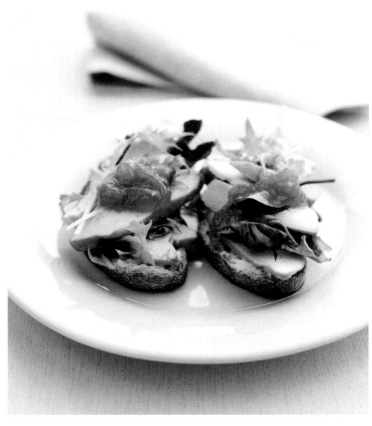

tuna salad bruschetta

PREPARATION TIME 5 MINUTES
COOKING TIME 2 MINUTES

At home, combine 95g can drained tuna in brine, 1 tablespoon low-fat mayonnaise, half of a small finely chopped red onion and 1 tablespoon coarsely chopped fresh flat-leaf parsley. At lunchtime, toast two slices ciabatta; divide tuna salad between slices.

smoked chicken and mango chutney bruschetta

PREPARATION TIME 5 MINUTES
COOKING TIME 2 MINUTES

At lunchtime, toast two slices ciabatta. Spread 1 teaspoon low-fat mayonnaise over both slices, then divide 100g thinly sliced smoked chicken, 10g mesclun and 1 tablespoon mango chutney between both slices.

NUTRITIONAL INFORMATION PER SERVING

6.5g total fat (1.6g saturated fat) **1304kJ (312 cal)**
37g carbohydrate **25.9g protein** 3g fibre

NUTRITIONAL INFORMATION PER SERVING

9.6g total fat (2.4g saturated fat) **1605kJ (384 cal)**
43.2g carbohydrate **30.8g protein** 2.8g fibre

MAINS

Old flavours in new partnerships create memorable mealtimes.

barley risotto with chicken and tarragon

PREPARATION TIME 15 MINUTES COOKING TIME 40 MINUTES SERVES 4

Pearl barley is barley that has had the husk removed, then been hulled and polished, much the same as rice.

1 tablespoon olive oil

500g chicken breast fillets, sliced thinly

3 cups (750ml) chicken stock

2 cups (500ml) water

1 medium brown onion (150g), chopped finely

1 clove garlic, crushed

2 medium leeks (700g), sliced thinly

¾ cup (150g) pearl barley

⅓ cup (80ml) dry white wine

1 cup (120g) frozen peas

2 tablespoons finely shredded fresh tarragon

1 Heat half of the oil in large saucepan; cook chicken, in batches, until browned lightly and cooked through. Cover to keep warm.

2 Meanwhile, combine stock and the water in large saucepan; bring to a boil. Reduce heat; simmer, covered.

3 Meanwhile, heat remaining oil in cleaned pan; cook onion, garlic and leek, stirring, until onion softens. Add barley; stir to combine with onion mixture. Add wine; cook, stirring, until almost evaporated. Stir in ½ cup of the simmering stock mixture; cook, stirring, over low heat until liquid is absorbed. Continue adding stock mixture, in ½-cup batches, stirring until absorbed after each addition. Total cooking time should be about 30 minutes or until barley is just tender.

4 Add chicken and peas to risotto; cook, stirring, until peas are just tender. Remove from heat; stir in tarragon.

NUTRITIONAL INFORMATION PER SERVING

9.7g total fat (1.9g saturated fat) **1584kJ (379 cal)** 31.6g carbohydrate **38g protein** 9.8g fibre

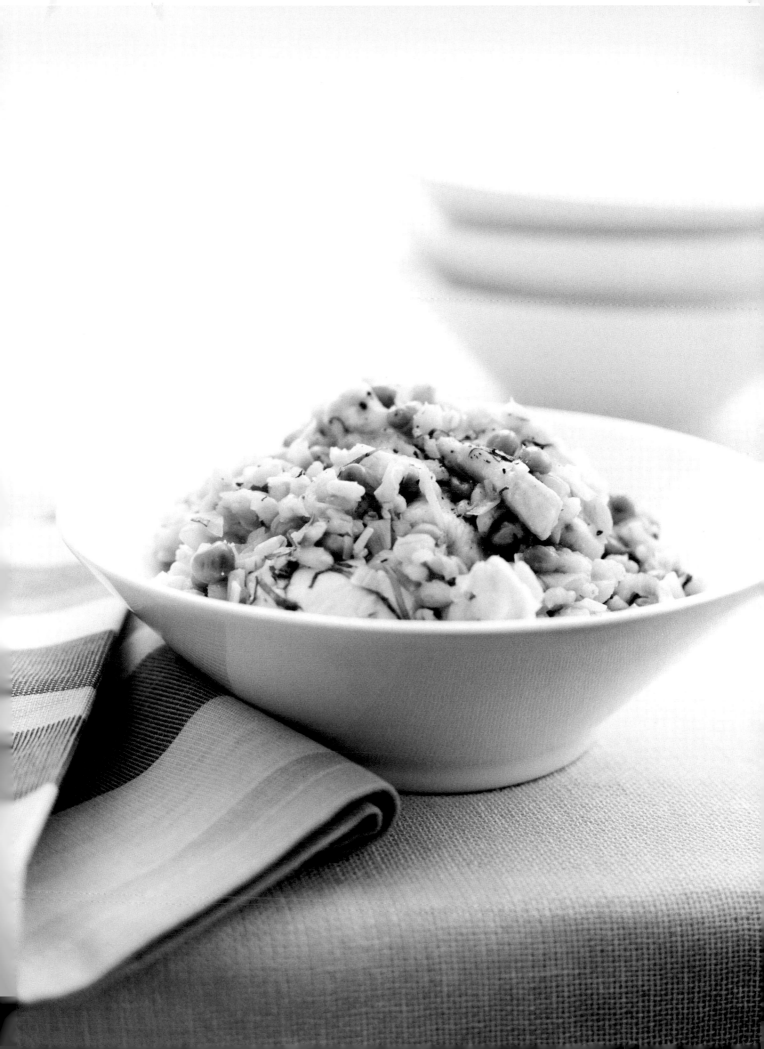

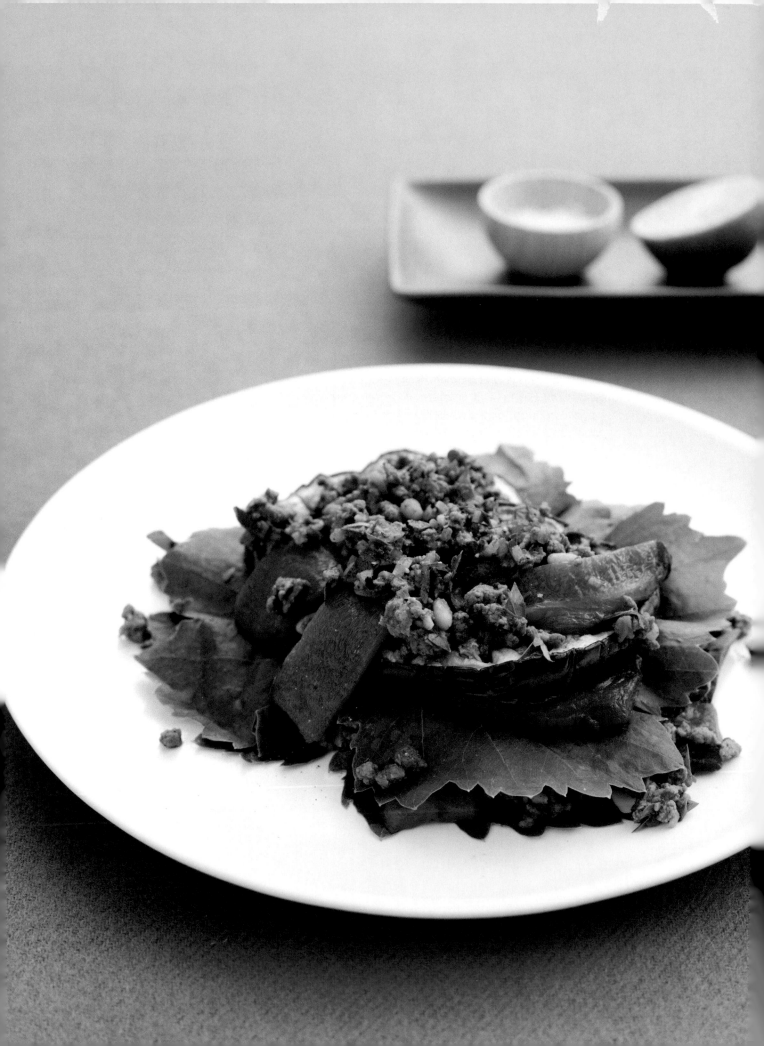

layered grapevine leaves, eggplant and lamb

PREPARATION TIME 20 MINUTES **COOKING TIME** 20 MINUTES **SERVES** 4

Baharat, an aromatic all-purpose spice blend, can be made with some or all of the following: mixed spice, black pepper, allspice, dried chilli flakes, paprika, coriander seeds, cinnamon, clove, sumac, nutmeg, cumin seeds and cardamom seeds. It is used throughout the Middle East; here, it is often sold as lebanese seven-spice, and can be found at Middle-Eastern food stores, some delicatessens and specialist food shops.

1 Quarter capsicums; remove seeds and membrane. Place capsicum, skin-side up, and eggplant on lightly oiled oven tray under preheated grill or in preheated hot oven until skin blisters. Cover capsicum with plastic wrap or paper for 5 minutes; peel away skin, then slice thinly.

2 Meanwhile, cook onion and garlic in heated lightly oiled large frying pan, stirring, until onion just softens. Add mince and spice; cook, stirring, until mince changes colour. Stir in combined brandy, paste and stock; bring to a boil. Reduce heat; simmer, uncovered, stirring, about 2 minutes or until liquid reduces by half. Remove from heat; stir in juice, nuts and parsley. Cover to keep warm.

3 Place vine leaves in large saucepan of boiling water, uncovered, for about 30 seconds or just until pliable; drain, in single layer, on absorbent paper.

4 Place one leaf on each plate; layer each leaf with one slice of eggplant, a few capsicum slices, ¼ cup mince mixture and another vine leaf. Repeat layering with remaining eggplant, capsicum and mince.

TIPS Make a substitute for baharat by combining 2 teaspoons paprika, 1 tablespoon ground cumin, 1 tablespoon ground coriander, 1 crushed clove and ½ teaspoon ground nutmeg.

If fresh vine leaves are unavailable, buy those preserved in brine and sold in Cryovac packages. Rinse thoroughly under cold water, then follow step 3 above, reducing time in the boiling water to 10 seconds.

2 large red capsicums (700g)

1 medium eggplant (300g), cut crossways into 12 slices

1 medium brown onion (150g), chopped finely

1 clove garlic, crushed

500g lamb mince

2 teaspoons baharat

1 tablespoon brandy

1 tablespoon tomato paste

½ cup (125ml) beef stock

1 tablespoon lime juice

1 tablespoon toasted pine nuts

1 cup coarsely chopped fresh flat-leaf parsley

8 fresh grapevine leaves

NUTRITIONAL INFORMATION PER SERVING

15.5g total fat (5.9g saturated fat) **1321kJ (316 cal)** 10.4g carbohydrate **31.1g protein** 5.6g fibre

Classic Italian
melt-in-the-mouth
morsels with a
faintly sweet flavour
heightened by herbs.

kumara gnocchi with rocket and basil pesto

PREPARATION TIME 45 MINUTES (PLUS REFRIGERATION TIME)
COOKING TIME 25 MINUTES **SERVES** 4

This gnocchi dough is very soft, so you'll need an extra half a cup of plain flour for the board when kneading and rolling to prevent it from sticking.

2 medium unpeeled kumara (800g)

4 small unpeeled desiree potatoes (480g)

1 cup (150g) plain flour

1 egg yolk

ROCKET AND BASIL PESTO

2 tablespoons olive oil

2 tablespoons finely grated parmesan cheese

1 clove garlic, quartered

2 tablespoons lemon juice

50g baby rocket leaves

1 cup firmly packed fresh basil leaves

1 Boil, steam or microwave kumara and potatoes, separately, until tender; drain. Peel when cool enough to handle; chop coarsely. Using wooden spoon, push kumara and potato through fine sieve into large bowl.

2 Stir flour and yolk into kumara mixture then knead dough gently on floured surface until mixture comes together. Divide dough into four portions; roll each portion into 40cm log, cut each log into 24 pieces. Roll each piece into a ball; roll balls, one at a time, along the inside tines of a floured fork, pressing gently on top of dough with index finger to form gnocchi shape (grooved on one side and dimpled on the other). Place gnocchi, in single layer, on lightly floured trays, cover; refrigerate 1 hour.

3 Place ingredients for rocket and basil pesto in blender or processor; process until smooth.

4 Cook gnocchi, in batches, uncovered, in large saucepan of boiling water about 3 minutes or until gnocchi float to surface. Remove gnocchi from pan with slotted spoon. Gently toss gnocchi in large bowl with pesto; serve topped with baby rocket leaves, if desired.

NUTRITIONAL INFORMATION PER SERVING

12.6g total fat (2.5g saturated fat) **1914kJ (458 cal)** 71.8g carbohydrate **13.4g protein** 8g fibre

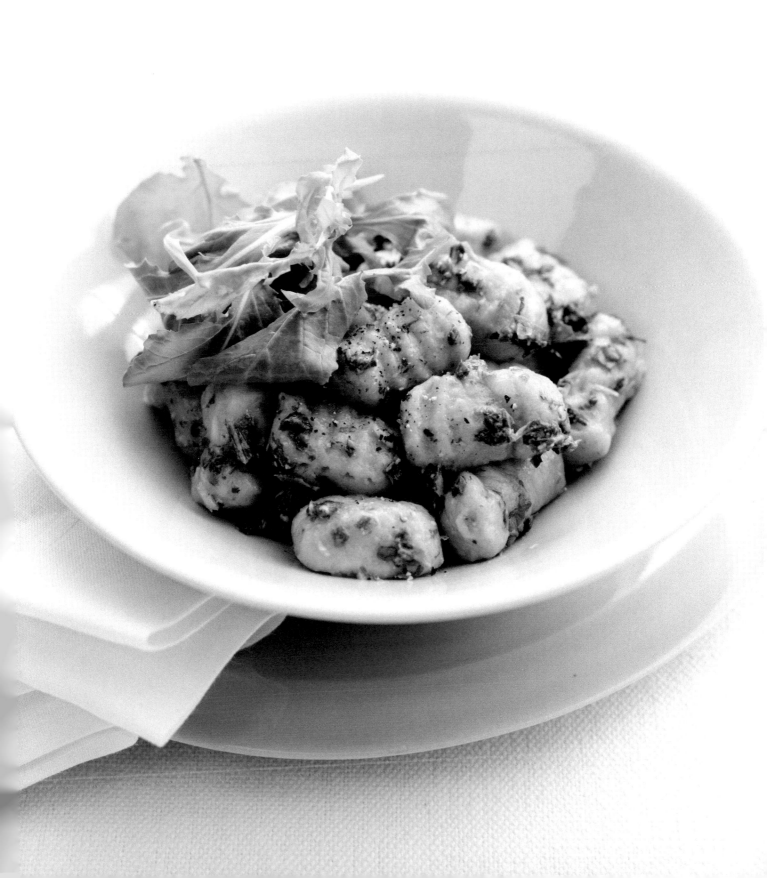

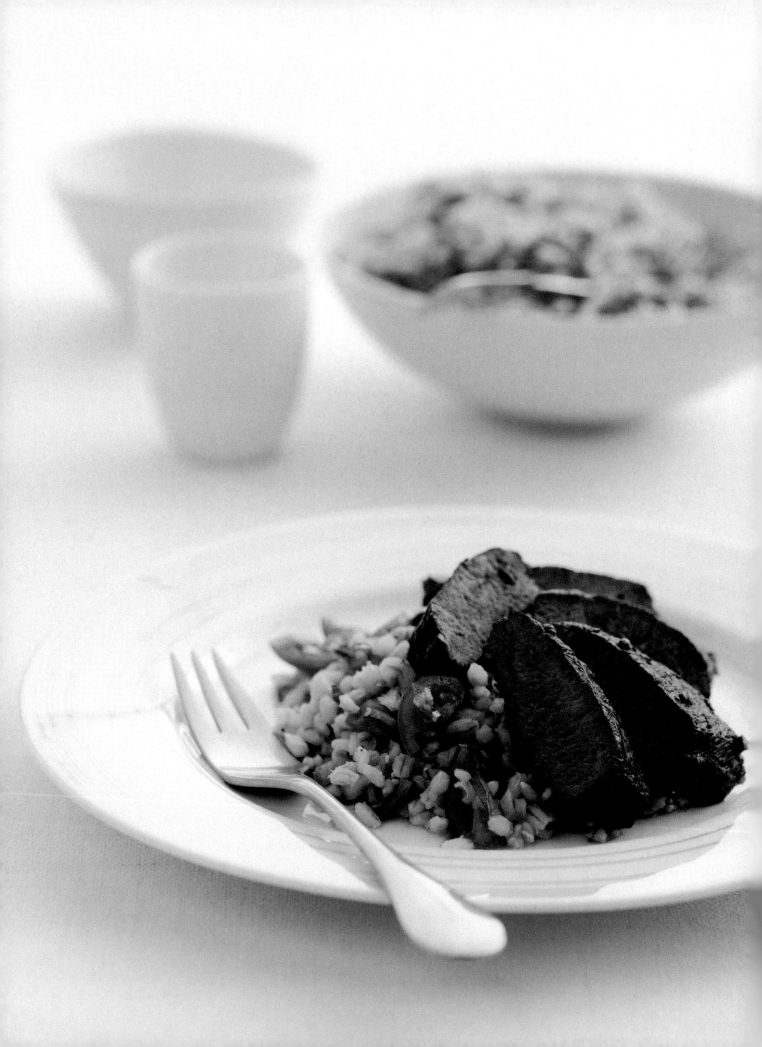

Simple and superb – lamb with a coating of spices from the Middle East, prepared ahead of time and cooked on the grill.

chilli coriander lamb with barley salad

PREPARATION TIME 20 MINUTES **COOKING TIME** 30 MINUTES
SERVES 4

1 Combine seeds, chilli and garlic in medium bowl, add lamb; toss lamb to coat in mixture. Cover; refrigerate until required.
2 Meanwhile, cook barley in large saucepan of boiling water, uncovered, about 20 minutes or until just tender; drain. Rinse under cold water; drain.
3 Cook lamb on heated lightly oiled grill plate (or grill or barbecue) until cooked as desired. Cover lamb; stand 5 minutes before slicing thickly.
4 Combine remaining ingredients in large bowl, add barley; toss gently to combine. Serve salad with lamb.

1 tablespoon coriander seeds, crushed lightly

½ teaspoon dried chilli flakes

2 cloves garlic, crushed

4 lamb backstraps (800g)

1 cup (200g) pearl barley

¼ teaspoon ground turmeric

⅓ cup coarsely chopped fresh mint

⅓ cup coarsely chopped fresh coriander

1 small red onion (100g), chopped finely

250g cherry tomatoes, quartered

¼ cup (60ml) lemon juice

2 teaspoons olive oil

NUTRITIONAL INFORMATION PER SERVING

10.9g total fat (3.8g saturated fat) **1822kJ (436 cal)** 33.8g carbohydrate **49.2g protein** 7.8g fibre

Pork partners well with fruit – try this sweet citrus glaze or experiment with other juices, such as apple, pear or mango.

orange-glazed pork cutlets with spinach and pecan salad

PREPARATION TIME 20 MINUTES **COOKING TIME** 20 MINUTES **SERVES 4**

½ cup (125ml) orange juice

¼ cup (55g) white sugar

2 cloves garlic, crushed

4 pork cutlets (950g), trimmed

SPINACH AND PECAN SALAD

150g baby spinach leaves

¼ cup (35g) toasted pecans, chopped coarsely

150g snow peas, trimmed, halved

4 medium oranges (960g)

CITRUS DRESSING

2 tablespoons orange juice

1 tablespoon lemon juice

½ teaspoon dijon mustard

½ teaspoon white sugar

2 teaspoons olive oil

1 Combine juice, sugar and garlic in small saucepan, bring to a boil. Reduce heat; simmer, without stirring, about 10 minutes or until glaze reduces to about ⅓ cup.

2 Brush cutlets both sides with glaze; cook, uncovered, in heated lightly oiled large frying pan about 10 minutes or until cooked as desired, brushing frequently with remaining glaze. Cover to keep warm.

3 Meanwhile, make spinach and pecan salad.

4 Place citrus dressing ingredients in screw-top jar; shake well. Pour dressing over salad; toss gently to combine. Serve salad with cutlets.

SPINACH AND PECAN SALAD Combine spinach, nuts and snow peas in large bowl. Segment peeled oranges over salad to catch juice; add segments to salad, toss gently to combine.

NUTRITIONAL INFORMATION PER SERVING

17g total fat (3.8g saturated fat) **1935kJ (463 cal)** 33.2g carbohydrate **44.1g protein** 6.4g fibre

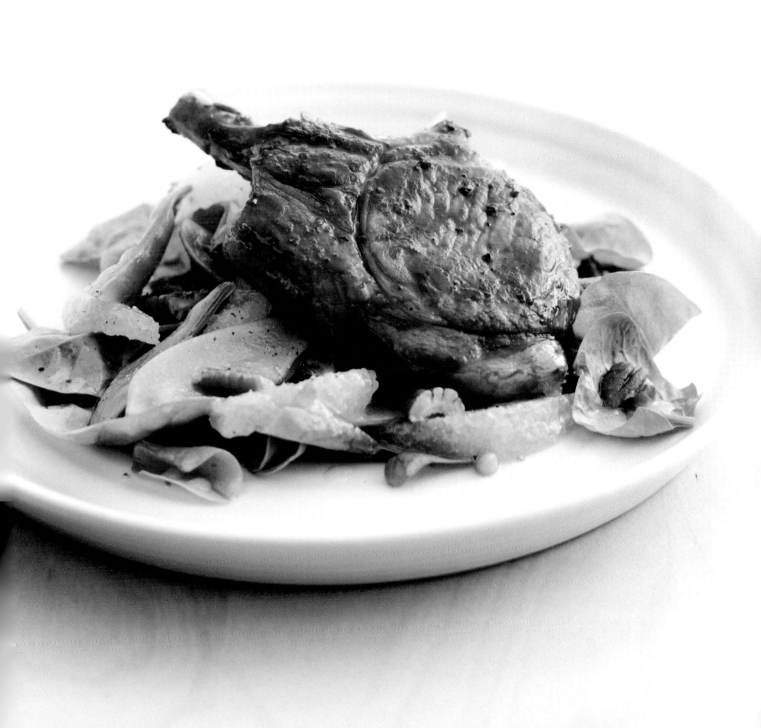

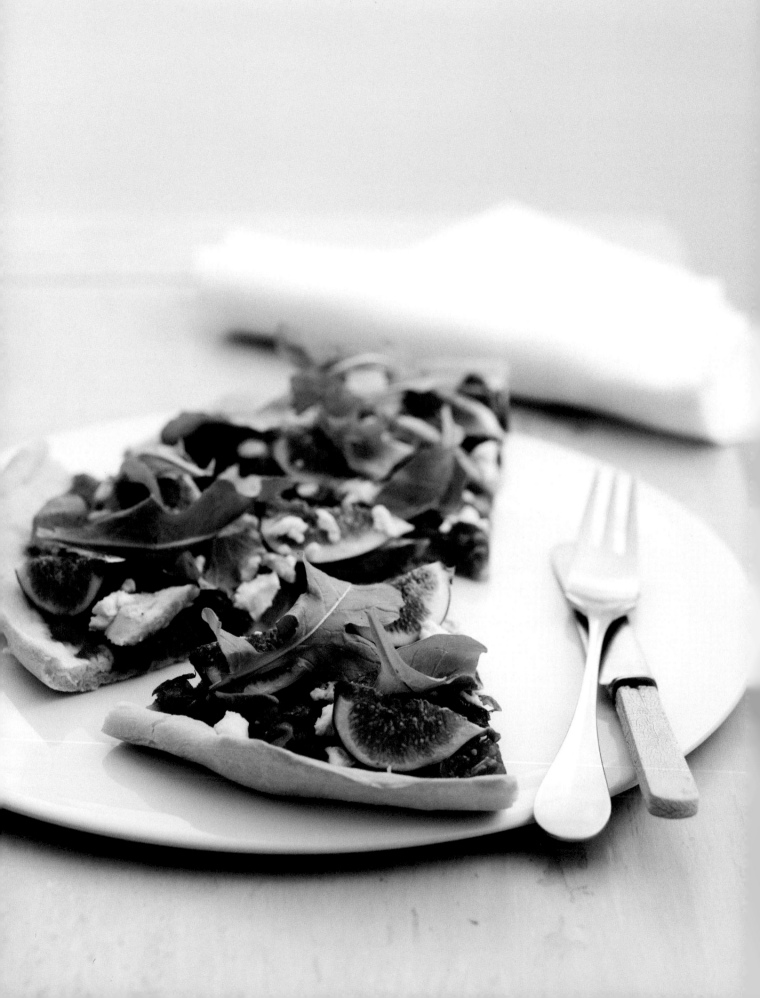

chicken, caramelised onion and fig pizza

PREPARATION TIME 30 MINUTES (PLUS STANDING TIME)
COOKING TIME 55 MINUTES **SERVES** 4

1 Make pizza dough. Make caramelised onion.
2 Preheat oven to moderately hot.
3 Cook chicken in heated lightly oiled small frying pan until cooked through. Cool 10 minutes; slice thinly.
4 Meanwhile, heat oil in small saucepan; cook garlic, stirring, until fragrant. Add undrained tomatoes; bring to a boil. Reduce heat; simmer, uncovered, about 15 minutes or until mixture thickens.
5 Sprinkle polenta onto two 30cm pizza trays. Halve pizza dough; roll each half on lightly floured surface to form 30cm-round pizza base. Place one base on each prepared tray; divide tomato sauce and caramelised onion between bases.
6 Cook pizzas, uncovered, in moderately hot oven about 10 minutes. Divide chicken, cheese and fig between pizzas; cook, uncovered, in moderately hot oven about 5 minutes or until bases are crisp. Sprinkle each with baby rocket leaves before serving.

PIZZA DOUGH Combine yeast, salt and flour in large bowl; gradually stir in the water and oil. Turn dough onto lightly floured surface; knead until smooth. Place dough in lightly oiled large bowl; cover tightly with plastic wrap then a tea towel. Stand in warm place about 45 minutes or until dough doubles in size. Knead dough on floured surface until smooth.
CARAMELISED ONION Heat oil in large frying pan; cook onion, stirring, until softened. Add sugar and vinegar; cook, stirring occasionally, about 15 minutes or until onion caramelises.

200g chicken breast fillet

2 teaspoons olive oil

2 cloves garlic, crushed

425g can crushed tomatoes

1 tablespoon polenta

100g firm goat cheese

4 large fresh figs (320g), quartered

50g baby rocket leaves

PIZZA DOUGH

2 teaspoons (7g) instant yeast

½ teaspoon salt

2½ cups (375g) plain flour

1 cup (250ml) warm water

2 teaspoons olive oil

CARAMELISED ONION

1 tablespoon olive oil

3 large brown onions (600g), sliced thinly

2 tablespoons brown sugar

2 tablespoons balsamic vinegar

NUTRITIONAL INFORMATION PER SERVING

16.2g total fat (4.4g saturated fat) **2663kJ (637 cal)** 92g carbohydrate **30.1g protein** 9.6g fibre

Pasta with effortless ingredients, assembled in minutes, is perfect for al fresco dining with good friends.

pappardelle with roasted tomato, spinach and ricotta

PREPARATION TIME 10 MINUTES **COOKING TIME** 25 MINUTES **SERVES** 4

A wide, ribbon-like pasta with scalloped sides, pappardelle is sometimes sold as lasagnette or even lasagne. Any wide, long pasta can be used for this recipe.

¼ cup (60ml) balsamic vinegar

3 cloves garlic, crushed

4 medium tomatoes (600g), cut into eight wedges

375g pappardelle

100g baby spinach leaves, trimmed

2 tablespoons olive oil

200g low-fat ricotta

1 Preheat oven to moderately hot.
2 Combine vinegar and garlic in small jug. Place tomato, in single layer, on oven tray; pour vinegar mixture over tomato. Roast, uncovered, in moderately hot oven about 25 minutes or until tomato is browned lightly and softened.
3 Meanwhile, cook pasta in large saucepan of boiling water, uncovered, until just tender.
4 Combine drained pasta, tomato, spinach and oil in large bowl. Break ricotta into approximately 3cm pieces; add to pasta mixture, toss gently to combine.

NUTRITIONAL INFORMATION PER SERVING

14.8g total fat (4.3g saturated fat) **2057kJ (492 cal)** 70.5g carbohydrate **17.8g protein** 7.7g fibre

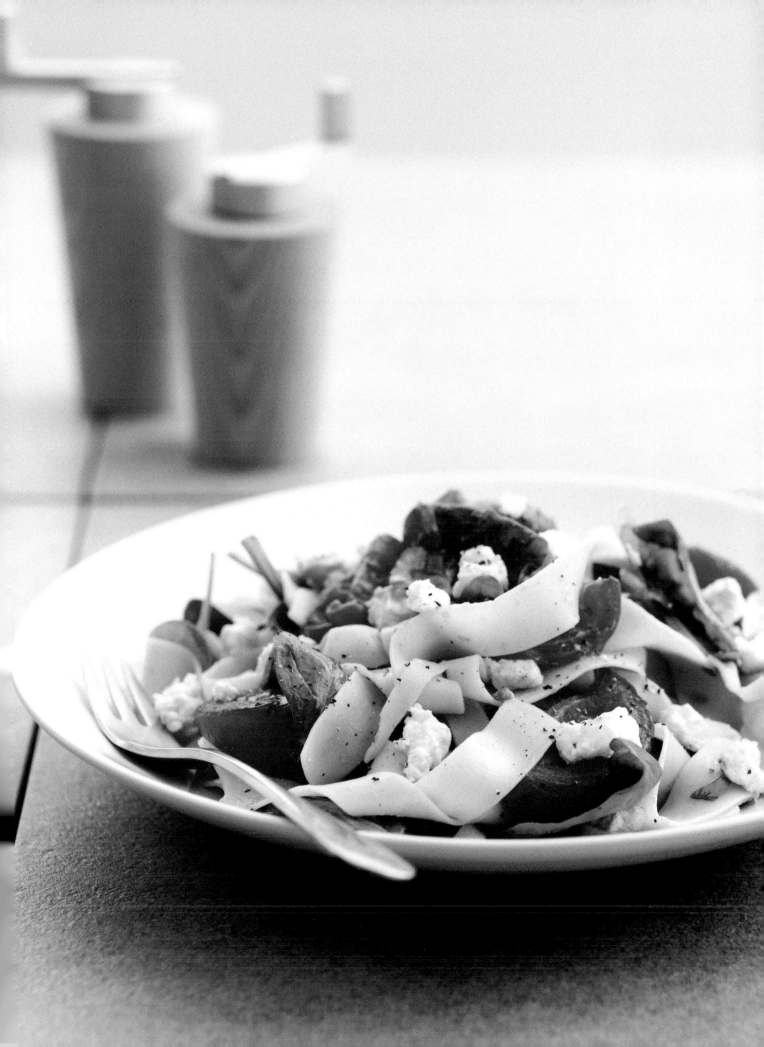

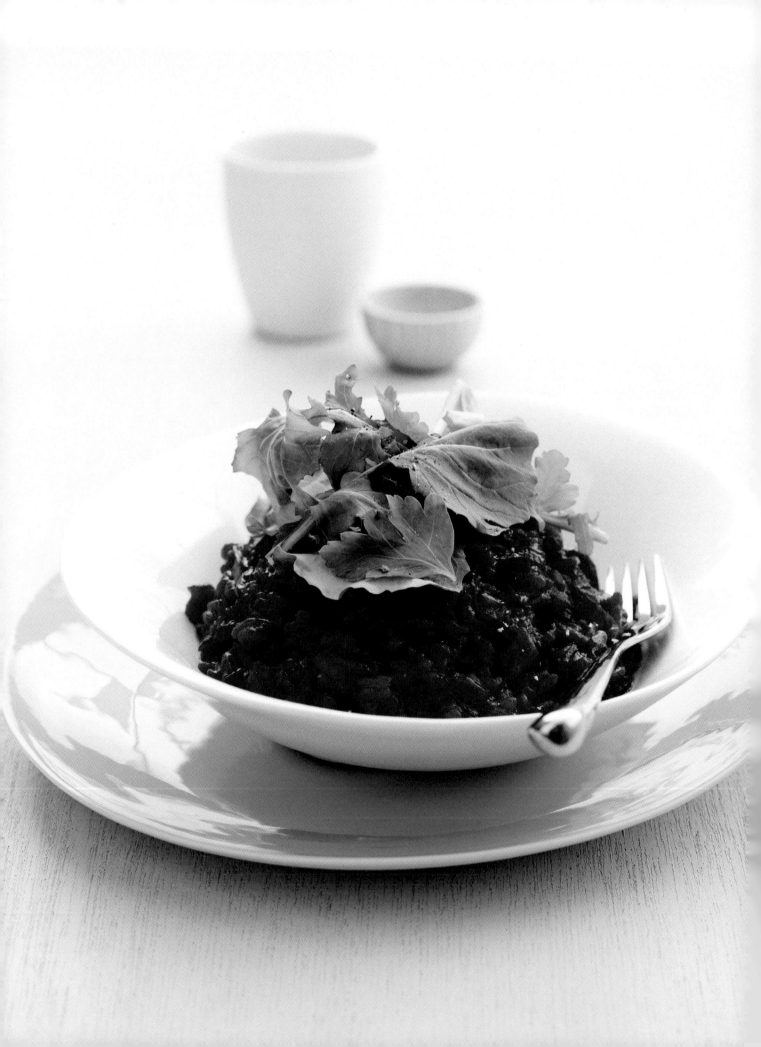

Look at me, look at me! – everything else on the table will pale in comparison to the splendour of this subtly sweet risotto.

beetroot risotto with rocket

PREPARATION TIME 30 MINUTES **COOKING TIME** 45 MINUTES
SERVES 4

1 Combine beetroot, stock and the water in large saucepan; bring to a boil. Reduce heat; simmer, uncovered.
2 Meanwhile, heat oil in large saucepan; cook onion and garlic, stirring, until onion softens. Add rice; stir rice to coat in onion mixture. Stir in 1 cup simmering beetroot mixture; cook, stirring, over low heat until liquid is absorbed. Continue adding beetroot mixture, in 1-cup batches, stirring, until liquid is absorbed after each addition. Total cooking time should be about 35 minutes or until rice is just tender; gently stir in cheese.
3 Serve beetroot risotto topped with combined rocket and parsley.

2 medium beetroot (350g), peeled, grated coarsely

3 cups (750ml) vegetable stock

3 cups (750ml) water

1 tablespoon olive oil

1 large brown onion (200g), chopped finely

2 cloves garlic, crushed

1½ cups (300g) arborio rice

¼ cup (20g) coarsely grated parmesan cheese

50g baby rocket leaves

1 tablespoon finely chopped fresh flat-leaf parsley

NUTRITIONAL INFORMATION PER SERVING

7.6g total fat (2.1g saturated fat) **1643kJ (393 cal)** 69.4g carbohydrate **11.5g protein** 4.1g fibre

Traditional to North Africa, a tagine is an aromatic casserole, usually cooked and served in an earthenware dish, also called a tagine.

pumpkin and split pea tagine

PREPARATION TIME 15 MINUTES **COOKING TIME** 40 MINUTES **SERVES** 4

1 cup (200g) green split peas

1 tablespoon olive oil

1 medium brown onion (150g), chopped finely

2 cloves garlic, crushed

2 teaspoons ground coriander

2 teaspoons ground cumin

2 teaspoons ground ginger

1 teaspoon sweet paprika

1 teaspoon ground allspice

1kg pumpkin, diced into 3cm pieces

425g can crushed tomatoes

1 cup (250ml) water

1 cup (250ml) vegetable stock

2 tablespoons honey

200g green beans, trimmed, chopped coarsely

¼ cup coarsely chopped fresh coriander

1 Cook split peas in medium saucepan of boiling water, uncovered, until just tender; drain. Rinse under cold water; drain.

2 Meanwhile, heat oil in large saucepan; cook onion, stirring, until softened. Add garlic and spices; cook, stirring, about 2 minutes or until fragrant. Add pumpkin; stir pumpkin to coat in spice mixture.

3 Stir in undrained tomatoes, the water and stock; bring to a boil. Reduce heat; simmer, uncovered, about 20 minutes or until pumpkin is just tender. Stir in honey then beans and split peas, reduce heat; simmer, uncovered, about 10 minutes or until beans are just tender. Remove from heat; stir in coriander. Serve with steamed couscous, if desired.

NUTRITIONAL INFORMATION PER SERVING

7g total fat (1.5g saturated fat) **1484kJ (355 cal)** 54.5g carbohydrate **19.1g protein** 11g fibre

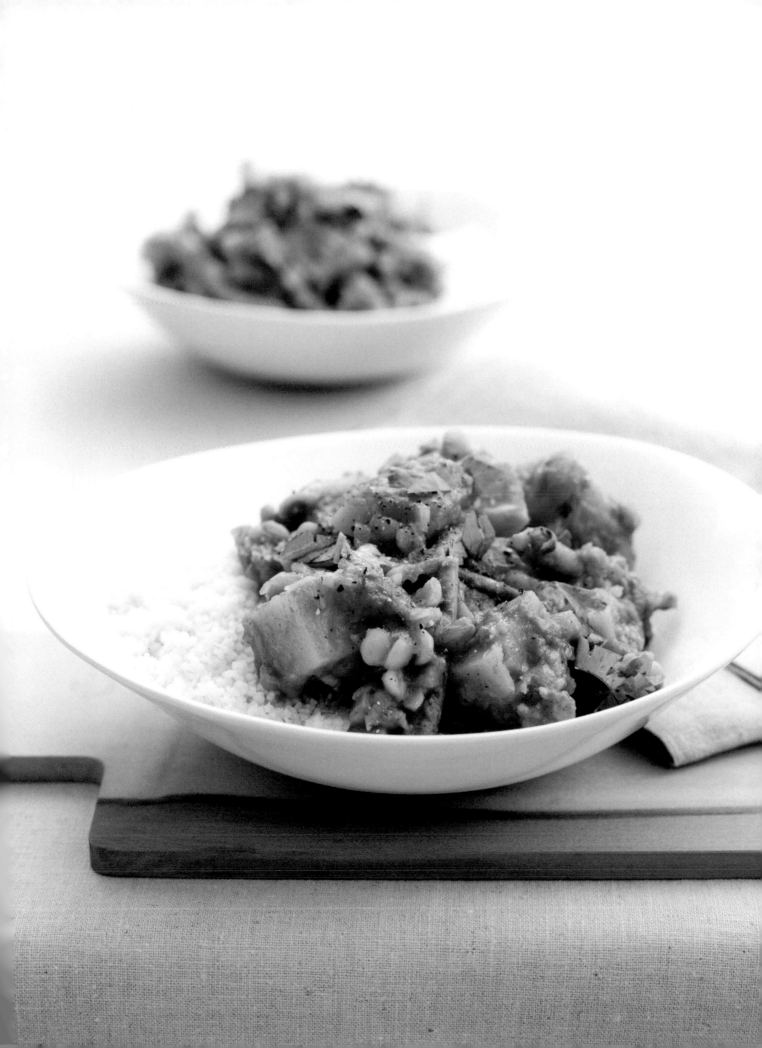

Let the good times
roll with this elegant
dinner party dish.

veal, mushroom and fennel rolls with horseradish mash

PREPARATION TIME 30 MINUTES **COOKING TIME** 35 MINUTES **SERVES** 4

1 tablespoon olive oil

2 cloves garlic, crushed

2 small fennel bulbs (400g), sliced thinly

3 flat mushrooms (240g), sliced thickly

½ cup (125ml) dry white wine

1½ cups (375ml) chicken stock

6 veal steaks (600g)

1 tablespoon finely chopped fresh flat-leaf parsley

HORSERADISH MASH

800g medium potatoes, chopped coarsely

2 tablespoons horseradish cream

¾ cup (180ml) hot skim milk

2 tablespoons finely chopped fresh flat-leaf parsley

1 Heat half of the oil in large frying pan; cook garlic and fennel, stirring, until fennel browns lightly. Add mushroom, half of the wine and ½ cup of the stock; bring to a boil. Reduce heat; simmer, uncovered, about 15 minutes or until liquid has evaporated. Cool 10 minutes.

2 Meanwhile, using meat mallet, gently pound veal steaks, one at a time, between pieces of plastic wrap until about 5mm thick; cut each piece in half crossways.

3 Divide fennel mixture among veal pieces; roll to enclose filling, securing each roll with a toothpick.

4 Make horseradish mash.

5 Heat remaining oil in large frying pan; cook rolls, uncovered, until cooked as desired. Cover to keep warm. Place remaining wine in same pan; bring to a boil, stirring. Boil 2 minutes then add remaining stock; bring to a boil, stirring. Boil, uncovered, 5 minutes.

6 Serve veal with mash and sauce, sprinkled with parsley.

HORSERADISH MASH Boil, steam or microwave potato; drain. Mash potato in large bowl; stir in horseradish and milk then parsley.

NUTRITIONAL INFORMATION PER SERVING

10.3g total fat (2.6g saturated fat) **1731kJ (414 cal)** 30.2g carbohydrate **44.1g protein** 6.6g fibre

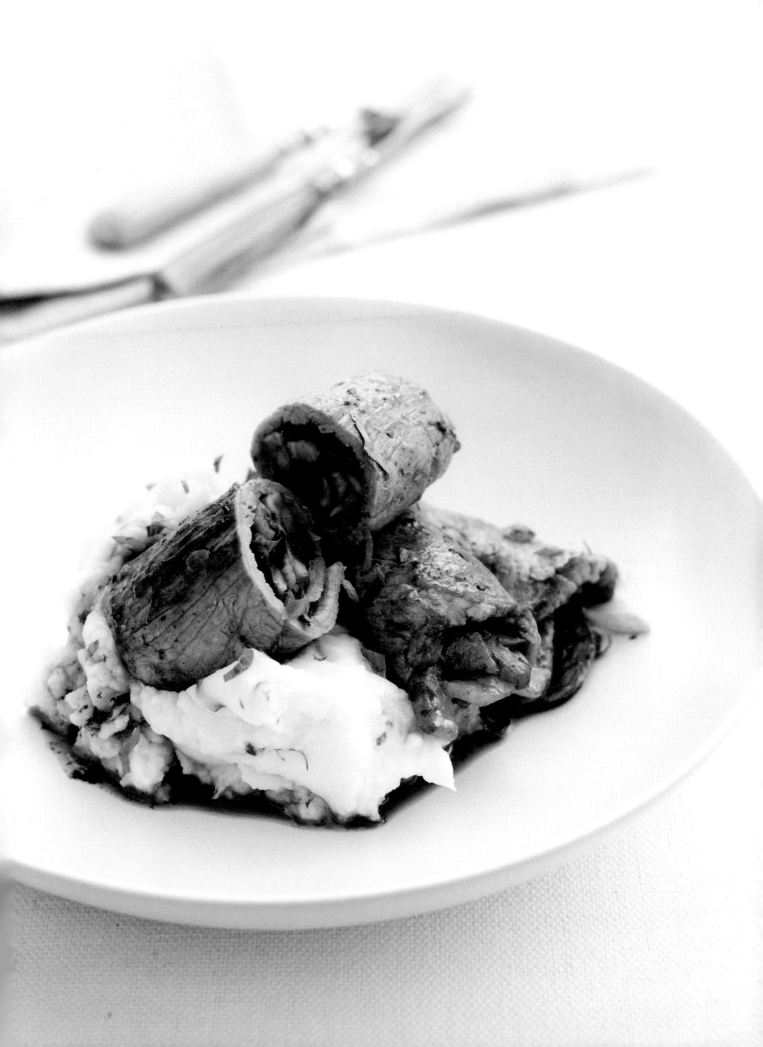

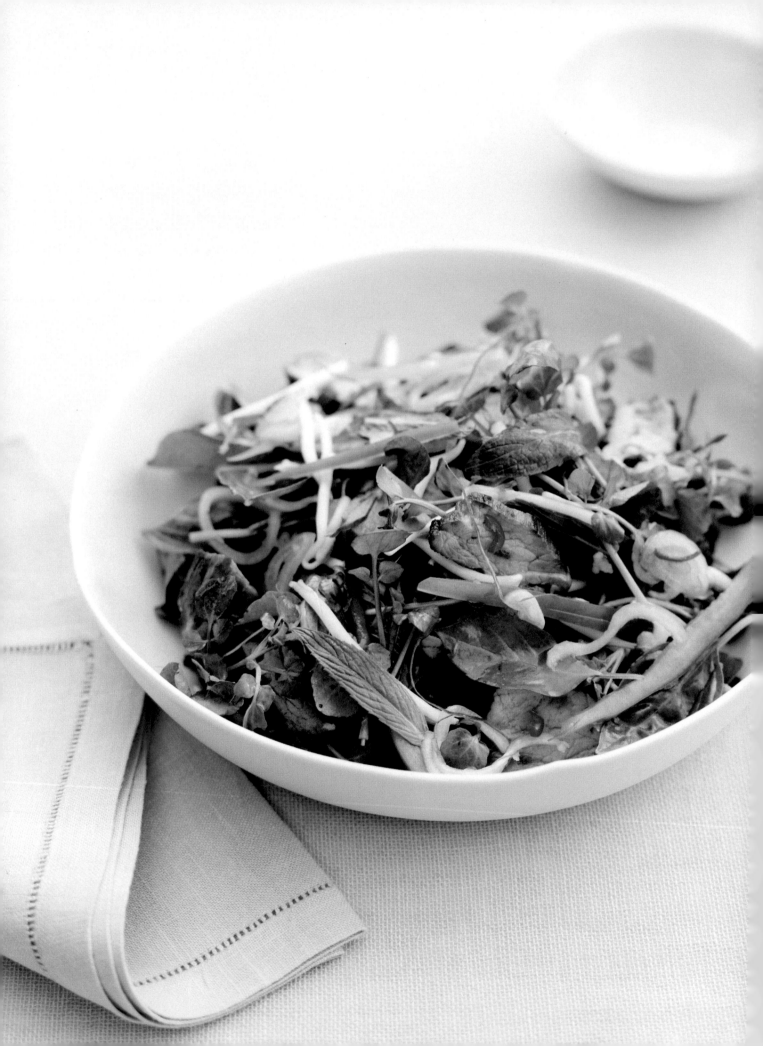

This crisp, fresh mix of thai flavours is a natural for outdoor entertaining.

thai pork salad with kaffir lime dressing

PREPARATION TIME 15 MINUTES **COOKING TIME** 15 MINUTES
SERVES 4

1 Cut pork fillets in half horizontally. Combine sugar, rind and oil in large bowl, add pork; toss pork to coat in mixture. Cook pork, in batches, in heated lightly oiled large frying pan, over medium heat, about 15 minutes or until cooked as desired. Cover pork; stand 5 minutes, then slice thinly.

2 Meanwhile, place kaffir lime dressing ingredients in screw-top jar; shake well.

3 Place pork in large bowl with remaining ingredients, add dressing; toss gently to combine.

600g pork fillets

2 tablespoons grated palm sugar

1 tablespoon finely grated lime rind

2 teaspoons peanut oil

350g watercress, trimmed

1 cup loosely packed fresh thai basil leaves

½ cup loosely packed fresh coriander leaves

½ cup loosely packed fresh mint leaves

1½ cups (120g) bean sprouts

1 medium green capsicum (200g), sliced thinly

KAFFIR LIME DRESSING

2 cloves garlic, crushed

3 shallots (75g), sliced thinly

1 fresh small red thai chilli, sliced thinly

3 fresh kaffir lime leaves, sliced thinly

¼ cup (60ml) lime juice

⅓ cup (80ml) fish sauce

2 teaspoons grated palm sugar

NUTRITIONAL INFORMATION PER SERVING

6.4g total fat (1.6g saturated fat) **1104kJ (264 cal)** 12.2g carbohydrate **38.8g protein** 5.8g fibre

Chop, dice, shake and slice a few hours ahead for a laid-back lunch.

shredded chicken salad

PREPARATION TIME 25 MINUTES **COOKING TIME** 10 MINUTES **SERVES** 4

500g chicken breast fillets

125g rice vermicelli

1 large carrot (180g), cut into matchsticks

1 medium red capsicum (200g), sliced thinly

1 medium green capsicum (200g), sliced thinly

1 lebanese cucumber (130g), seeded, sliced thinly

1 fresh long red chilli, sliced thinly

1 cup coarsely shredded fresh mint

¼ cup (35g) toasted unsalted peanuts, chopped coarsely

LIME AND PALM SUGAR DRESSING

¼ cup (60ml) lime juice

¼ cup (65g) grated palm sugar

¼ cup (60ml) fish sauce

1 Place lime and palm sugar dressing ingredients in screw-top jar; shake well.
2 Place chicken and half of the dressing in medium saucepan with barely enough boiling water to cover chicken; bring to a boil. Reduce heat; simmer, uncovered, about 10 minutes or until chicken is cooked through. Cool chicken in poaching liquid 10 minutes; discard liquid (or reserve for another use). Using two forks, shred chicken finely.
3 Meanwhile, place vermicelli in large heatproof bowl; cover with boiling water. Stand until just tender; drain. Rinse under cold water; drain.
4 Place chicken and vermicelli in large bowl with carrot, capsicums, cucumber, chilli, mint and remaining dressing; toss gently to combine. Divide salad among plates; top with nuts.

NUTRITIONAL INFORMATION PER SERVING

7.8g total fat (1.3g saturated fat) **1613kJ (386 cal)** 43.1g carbohydrate **35.6g protein** 4.6g fibre

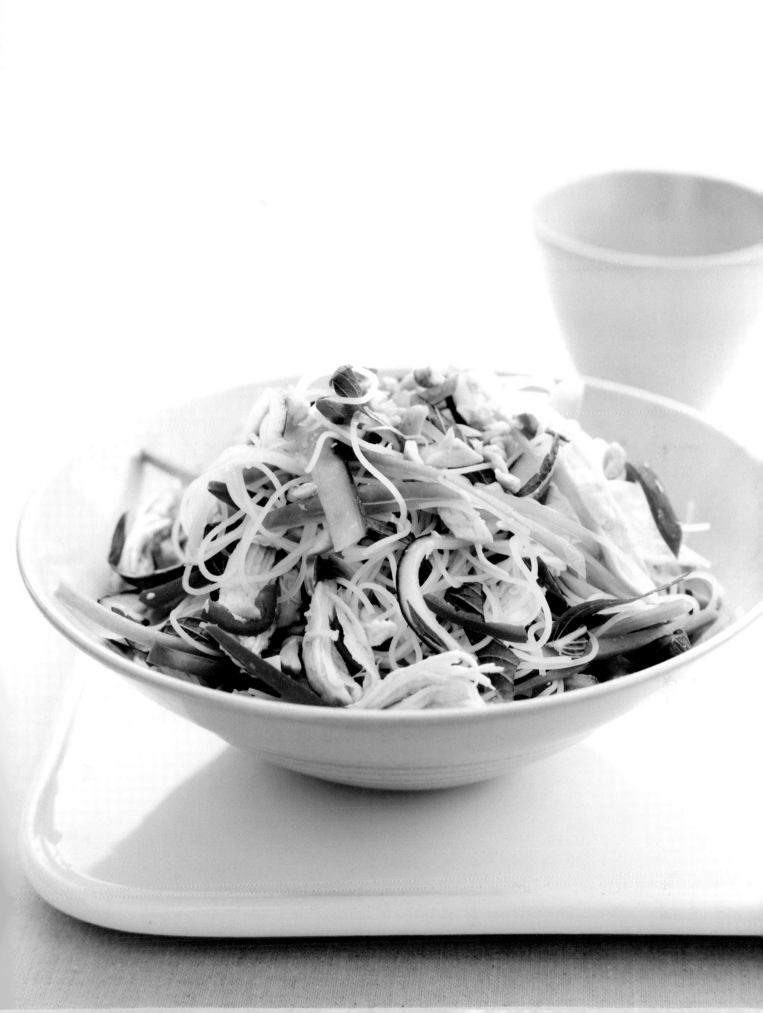

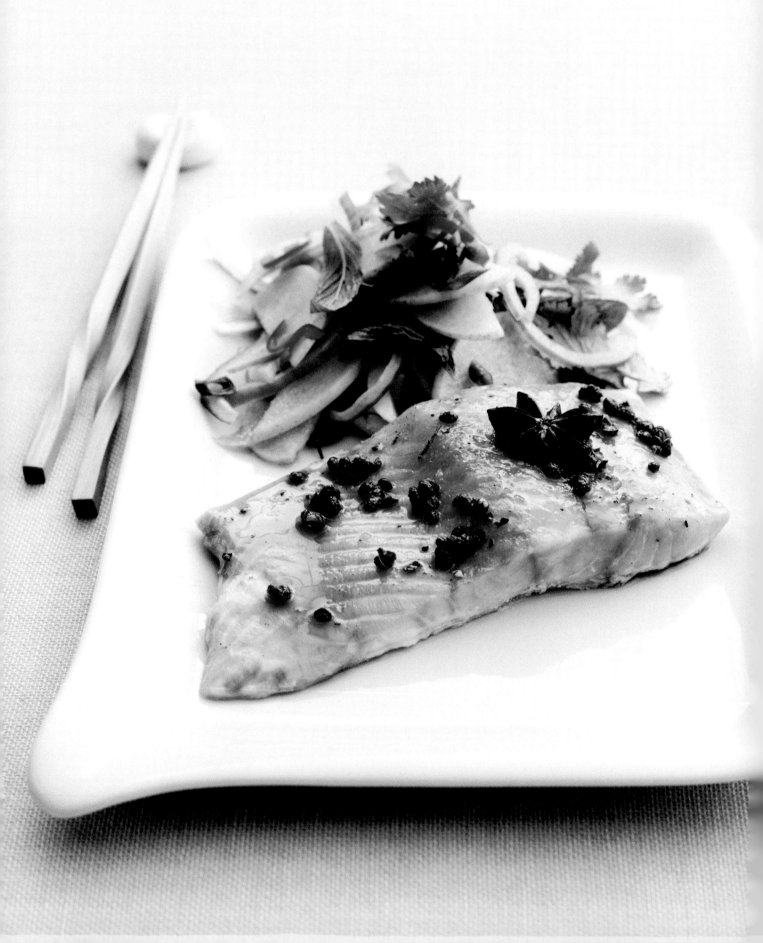

Let the exotic ingredients in this easy-to-prepare dish take you beyond your culinary comfort zone.

asian-spiced salmon with nashi, mint and coriander salad

PREPARATION TIME 20 MINUTES **COOKING TIME** 20 MINUTES **SERVES** 4

If nashi are not available, substitute with crisp green apples.

1 Preheat oven to moderate.
2 Dry-fry spices in small frying pan until fragrant. Add sauce and honey; bring to a boil. Reduce heat; simmer, uncovered, 2 minutes.
3 Line large shallow baking dish with foil, extending foil 5cm above long sides of dish; coat lightly with cooking-oil spray. Place fish on foil; brush both sides with spice mixture. Bake, uncovered, in moderate oven about 15 minutes or until cooked as desired.
4 Meanwhile, place sesame soy dressing ingredients in screw-top jar; shake well.
5 Place remaining ingredients in large bowl, add dressing; toss gently to combine. Serve salad with fish.

2 teaspoons sichuan peppercorns, crushed

2 star anise

1 tablespoon soy sauce

2 tablespoons honey

cooking-oil spray

4 salmon fillets (800g)

2 medium nashi (400g), sliced thinly

1 fresh long red chilli, sliced thinly

1 medium red onion (170g), sliced thinly

2 green onions, sliced thinly

¾ cup loosely packed fresh mint leaves

¾ cup loosely packed fresh coriander leaves

SESAME SOY DRESSING

2 tablespoons soy sauce

¼ cup (60ml) mirin

2 teaspoons caster sugar

¼ teaspoon sesame oil

NUTRITIONAL INFORMATION PER SERVING

17.5g total fat (3.7g saturated fat) **1864kJ (446 cal)** 26.7g carbohydrate **45.5g protein** 4g fibre

Use the softened, salty rind of preserved lemon to add a tangy intensity to this dish.

moroccan blue-eye kebabs with almond and lemon couscous

PREPARATION TIME 25 MINUTES (PLUS REFRIGERATION TIME)
COOKING TIME 10 MINUTES **SERVES** 4

You will need to soak eight 25cm bamboo skewers in water for at least an hour before using to prevent them from splintering or scorching.

½ cup finely chopped
fresh coriander

2 cloves garlic, crushed

2 tablespoons olive oil

2 fresh small red thai chillies,
chopped finely

¼ cup (60ml) lemon juice

800g skinless blue-eye fillets,
diced into 3cm pieces

1½ cups (375ml) chicken stock

1½ cups (300g) couscous

½ cup firmly packed fresh
coriander leaves

1 tablespoon finely chopped
preserved lemon

¼ cup (35g) toasted
slivered almonds

1 Combine chopped coriander, garlic, oil, chilli and juice in small bowl. Place half of the coriander mixture in large bowl, add fish; toss fish to coat in mixture. Thread fish onto skewers; place kebabs on tray. Cover; refrigerate 45 minutes.

2 Cook kebabs on heated lightly oiled grill plate (or grill or barbecue) about 5 minutes or until cooked as desired.

3 Meanwhile, bring stock to a boil in small saucepan; remove from heat. Add couscous to stock, cover; stand about 5 minutes or until liquid is absorbed, fluffing with fork occasionally. Add remaining coriander mixture, coriander leaves, lemon and nuts; toss gently to combine. Serve couscous with kebabs.

NUTRITIONAL INFORMATION PER SERVING

16g total fat (2.2g saturated fat) **2391kJ (572 cal)** 59.2g carbohydrate **46.6 protein** 2.6g fibre

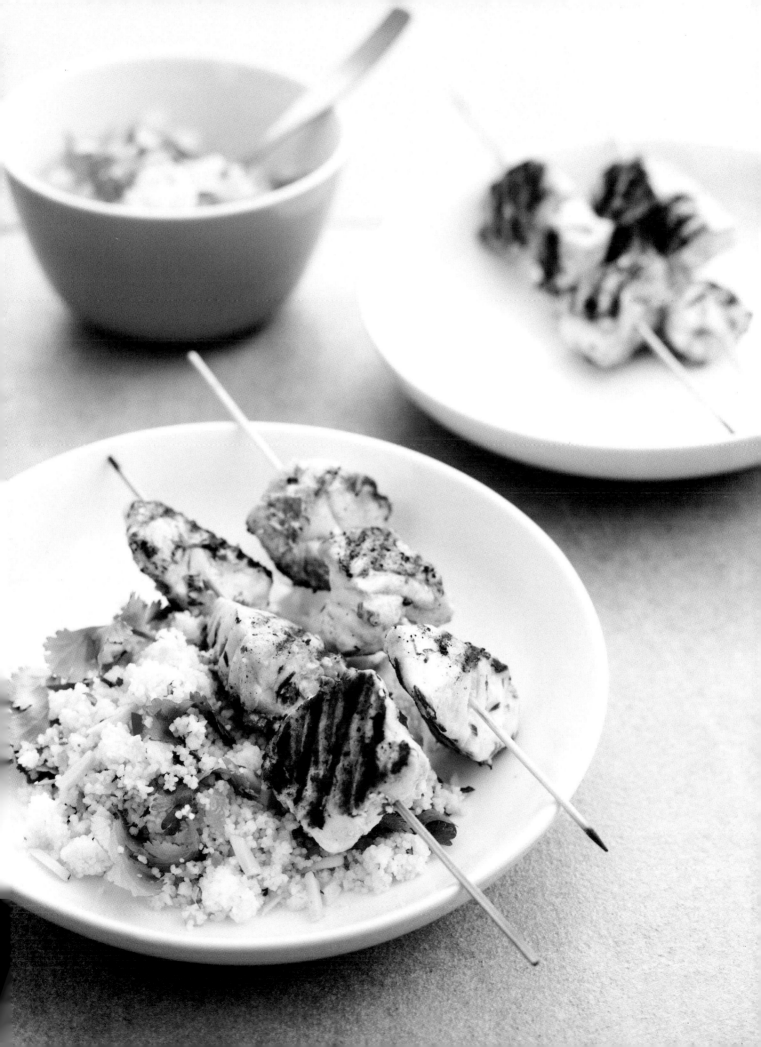

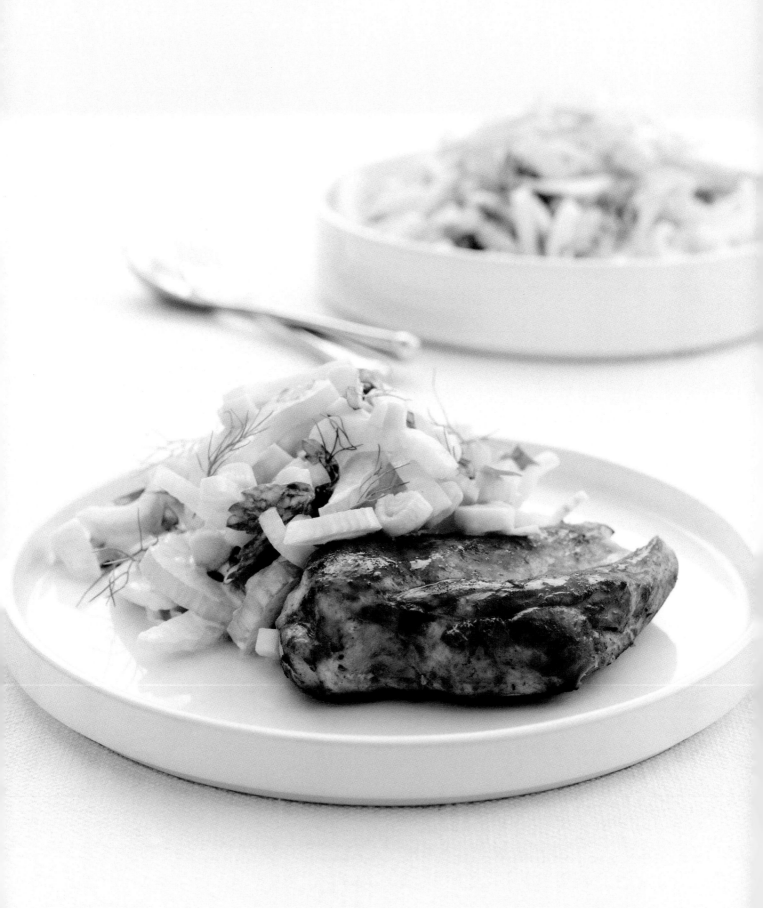

With a bit of a bite, fennel and mustard reinvent the classic chicken and salad combo.

honey dijon chicken with creamy celery and fennel slaw

PREPARATION TIME 20 MINUTES **COOKING TIME** 30 MINUTES
SERVES 4

1 Combine honey and mustard in small bowl. Brush chicken both sides with half of the honey mixture; cook, in batches, in heated lightly oiled large frying pan about 15 minutes or until cooked through, brushing with remaining honey mixture.
2 Meanwhile, make creamy fennel and celery slaw.
3 Serve chicken with slaw, sprinkled with reserved fennel tips.

CREAMY FENNEL AND CELERY SLAW Trim fennel, reserving about 1 tablespoon of the tips (discard the rest). Slice fennel thinly; combine with celery and parsley in large bowl. Combine remaining ingredients in small bowl, pour over slaw mixture; toss gently to combine.

2 tablespoons honey

2 teaspoons dijon mustard

4 single chicken breast fillets (680g)

CREAMY FENNEL
AND CELERY SLAW

2 medium fennel bulbs (600g)

3 trimmed celery stalks (300g), sliced thinly

¼ cup coarsely chopped fresh flat-leaf parsley

2 teaspoons dijon mustard

2 tablespoons lemon juice

2 tablespoons light sour cream

2 cloves garlic, crushed

¼ cup (75g) low-fat mayonnaise

NUTRITIONAL INFORMATION PER SERVING

8.8g total fat (2.9g saturated fat) **1371kJ (328 cal)** 21.2g carbohydrate **40.8g protein** 4.9g fibre

Seafood in asian greens, tied up with string… this will be one of your favourite things.

ocean trout in baby bok choy parcels

PREPARATION TIME 20 MINUTES (PLUS STANDING TIME)
COOKING TIME 15 MINUTES **SERVES** 4

Wash the bok choy carefully. It's important to remove all the dirt hidden among the leaves without actually separating any of the leaves from the base, thus leaving each vegetable intact.

4 dried shiitake mushrooms

2 green onions, chopped finely

3cm piece fresh ginger (15g), grated

5cm stick (10g) finely chopped fresh lemon grass

2 cloves garlic, crushed

1 teaspoon sambal oelek

2 tablespoons soy sauce

4 ocean trout fillets (600g)

4 large baby bok choy (600g)

1½ cups (300g) jasmine rice

GINGER DRESSING

2cm piece fresh ginger (10g), grated

2 tablespoons rice wine vinegar

1 tablespoon vegetable oil

1 teaspoon sesame oil

2 tablespoons mirin

1 tablespoon soy sauce

1 Place mushrooms in small heatproof bowl, cover with boiling water, stand 20 minutes; drain. Discard stems; chop caps finely.

2 Meanwhile, combine ginger dressing ingredients in screw-top jar; shake well.

3 Combine mushroom, onion, ginger, lemon grass, garlic, sambal and sauce in small bowl; divide mushroom mixture among flesh side of fish fillets. Carefully insert one fillet, mushroom-side up, inside leaves of each bok choy; wrap leaves around fillet then tie parcels with kitchen string.

4 Place parcels in large steamer fitted over large saucepan of boiling water; steam, covered, about 10 minutes or until fish is cooked as desired.

5 Meanwhile, cook rice in large saucepan of boiling water, uncovered, until rice is just tender; drain. Divide rice among plates; top with parcels, drizzle with dressing.

NUTRITIONAL INFORMATION PER SERVING

12.3g total fat (2.2g saturated fat) **2195kJ (525 cal)** 64.6g carbohydrate **37.1g protein** 3.6g fibre

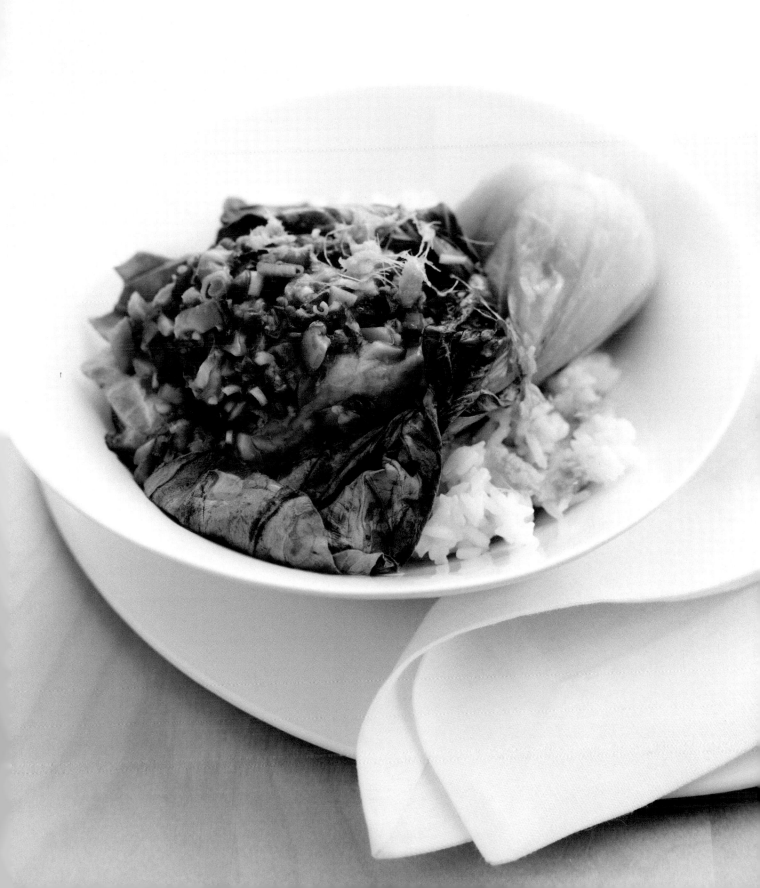

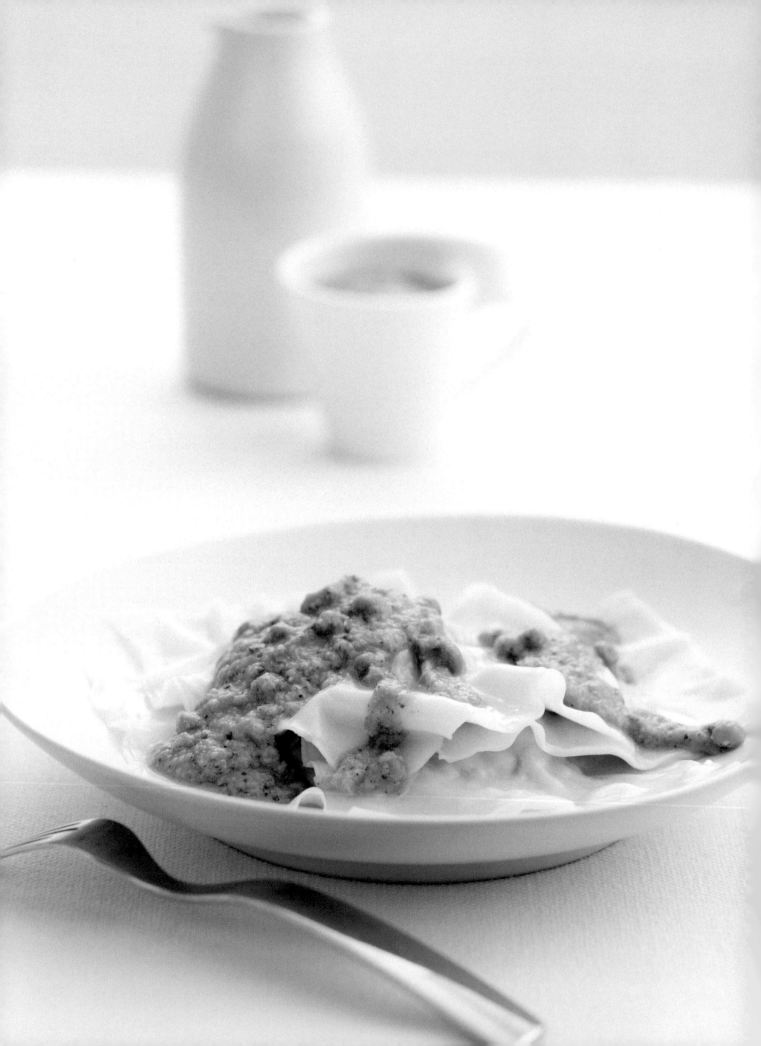

Wonton wrappers form the pasta packaging for a fabulous filling.

prawn ravioli with mint and pea puree

PREPARATION TIME 40 MINUTES **COOKING TIME** 15 MINUTES
SERVES 4

1 Bring chicken stock to a boil in medium saucepan. Add peas, mint and butter; return to a boil. Reduce heat; simmer, uncovered, about 5 minutes or until peas are soft. Cool 10 minutes; blend or process with garlic until smooth.

2 Meanwhile, shell and devein prawns; chop half of the prawns coarsely. Blend or process remaining whole prawns with egg white, sauce and half of the juice until mixture is almost smooth. Combine in large bowl with chopped prawn and chilli.

3 Centre 1 level tablespoon of the prawn mixture on one wrapper; brush around edges with water. Top with another wrapper; press edges together to seal. Repeat with remaining prawn mixture and wrappers; you will have 20 ravioli. Cook ravioli, in batches, in large saucepan of boiling water, uncovered, until ravioli float to the surface and are cooked.

4 Meanwhile, return pea puree to same medium saucepan, add extra peas and remaining juice; stir over heat until peas are just tender.

5 Divide drained ravioli among plates; top with pea puree.

1¼ cups (310ml) chicken stock

2½ cups (300g)) frozen peas

½ cup loosely packed fresh mint leaves

40g butter

1 clove garlic, crushed

1kg uncooked medium king prawns

1 egg white

1 tablespoon sweet chilli sauce

2 tablespoons lemon juice

1 long green chilli, chopped finely

40 wonton wrappers

¼ cup (30g) frozen peas, extra

NUTRITIONAL INFORMATION PER SERVING

10.8g total fat (6g saturated fat) **1613kJ (386 cal)** 34g carbohydrate **37.3g protein** 6.7g fibre

koshari

PREPARATION TIME 15 MINUTES **COOKING TIME** 45 MINUTES **SERVES** 4

Various combinations of rice and lentils are eaten throughout the Middle East and India, with perhaps the two most well-known versions being Lebanese mujadara and Indian kitcheree. Our Egyptian take on this homely dish, however, adds delicious "oomph" to the rice-lentil theme with its fragrantly spicy caramelised onion and piquant chilli sauce.

2 cups (400g) brown lentils

¾ cup (150g) white long-grain rice

1 cup coarsely chopped fresh flat-leaf parsley

CARAMELISED ONION

2 tablespoons olive oil

5 large brown onions (1kg), sliced thinly

1½ teaspoons ground allspice

1 teaspoon ground coriander

2 teaspoons white sugar

TOMATO CHILLI SAUCE

2 teaspoons olive oil

3 cloves garlic, crushed

½ teaspoon ground cumin

½ teaspoon dried chilli flakes

⅓ cup (80ml) white vinegar

415ml can tomato juice

1 Make caramelised onion. Make tomato chilli sauce.
2 Meanwhile, cook lentils in medium saucepan of boiling water, uncovered, until just tender; drain.
3 Cook rice in medium saucepan of boiling water, uncovered, until just tender; drain.
4 Remove half of the caramelised onion from pan, reserve. Add lentils and rice to pan, stirring, until heated through. Remove from heat; stir in half of the parsley.
5 Divide koshari among bowls; top with reserved caramelised onion, remaining parsley and tomato chilli sauce.

CARAMELISED ONION Heat oil in large frying pan; cook onion, allspice and coriander, stirring, until onion softens. Add sugar; cook, uncovered, stirring occasionally, about 30 minutes or until onion caramelises.

TOMATO CHILLI SAUCE Heat oil in small saucepan; cook garlic, cumin and chilli, stirring, until fragrant. Add vinegar and juice; bring to a boil. Boil, uncovered, 2 minutes.

NUTRITIONAL INFORMATION PER SERVING

13.9g total fat (2g saturated fat) **2416kJ (578 cal)** 83.3g carbohydrate **31.3g protein** 18.8g fibre

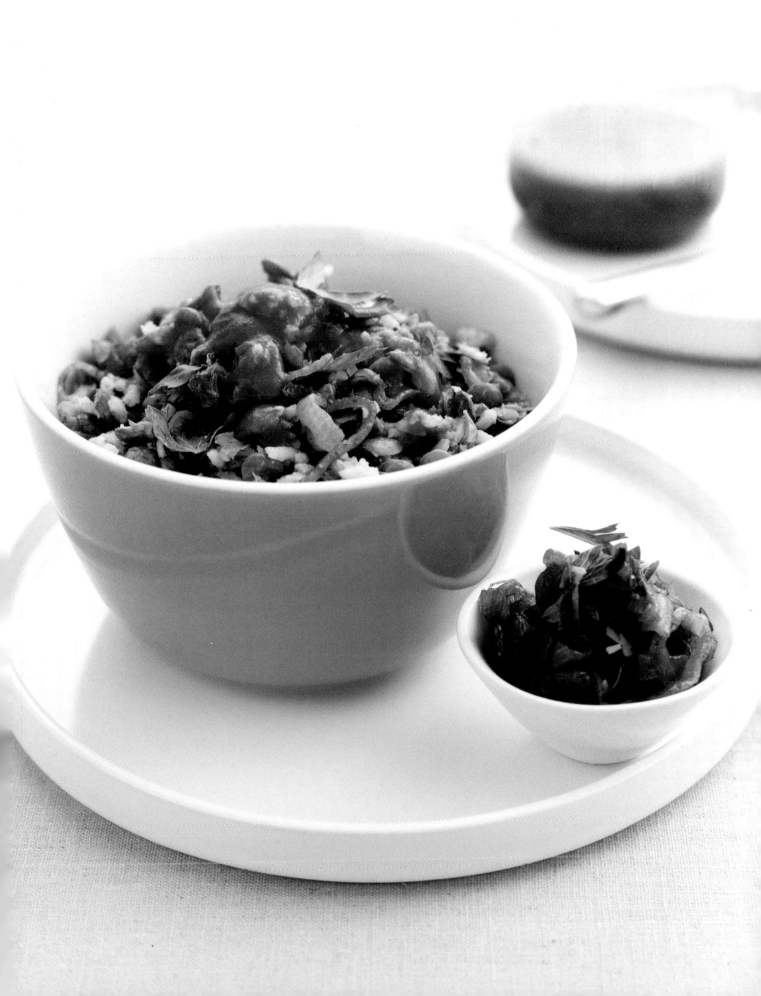

The delight of this
dish is its simplicity
- confident colours and
strong, clear flavours.

grilled snapper with spicy tomato sauce

PREPARATION TIME 15 MINUTES **COOKING TIME** 15 MINUTES **SERVES** 4

2 tablespoons olive oil

3 cloves garlic, crushed

3 shallots (75g), chopped finely

425g can diced tomatoes

1 tablespoon dry sherry

1 tablespoon soy sauce

1 teaspoon sambal oelek

2 teaspoons white sugar

4 snapper fillets (800g)

75g baby spinach leaves

2 teaspoons red wine vinegar

1 Heat half of the oil in small frying pan; cook garlic and shallots, stirring, about 1 minute or until shallots soften. Stir in undrained tomatoes, sherry, sauce, sambal and sugar; bring to a boil. Reduce heat; simmer, uncovered, about 10 minutes or until liquid has reduced by half.

2 Meanwhile, cook fish, uncovered, in heated lightly oiled large frying pan about 10 minutes or until cooked as desired.

3 Place spinach in medium bowl with combined vinegar and remaining oil; toss gently to combine. Serve fish with spicy sauce and spinach salad.

NUTRITIONAL INFORMATION PER SERVING

12.7g total fat (2.5g saturated fat) **1325kJ (317 cal)** 6.3g carbohydrate **42.5g protein** 2.3g fibre

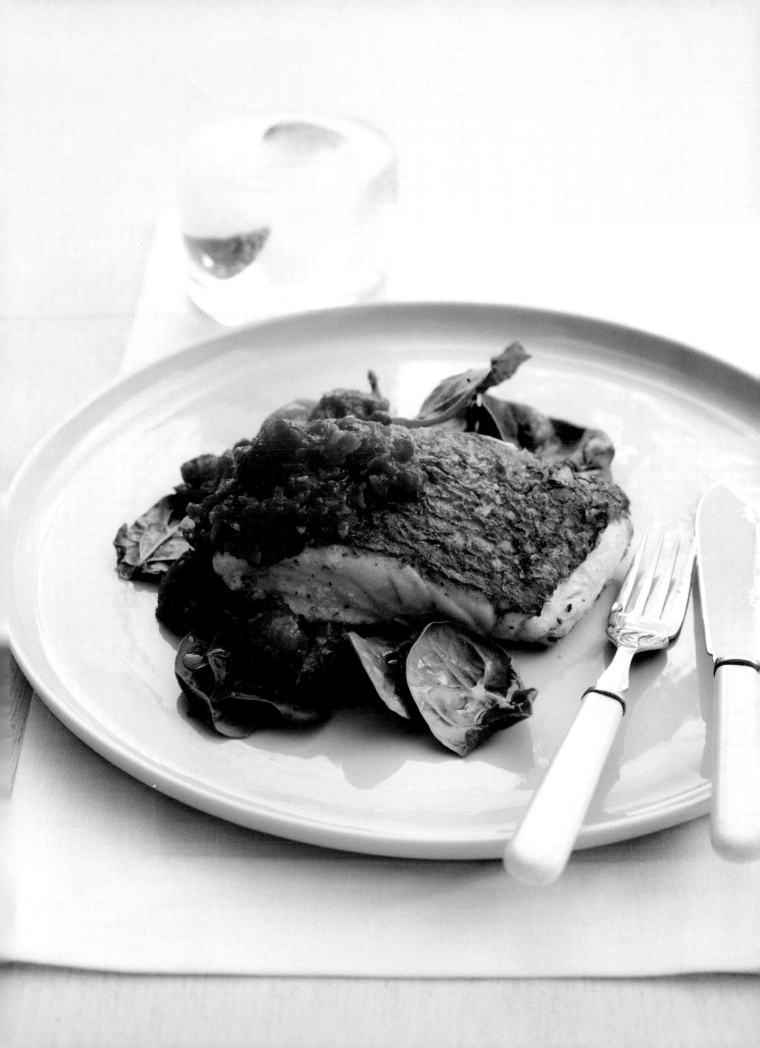

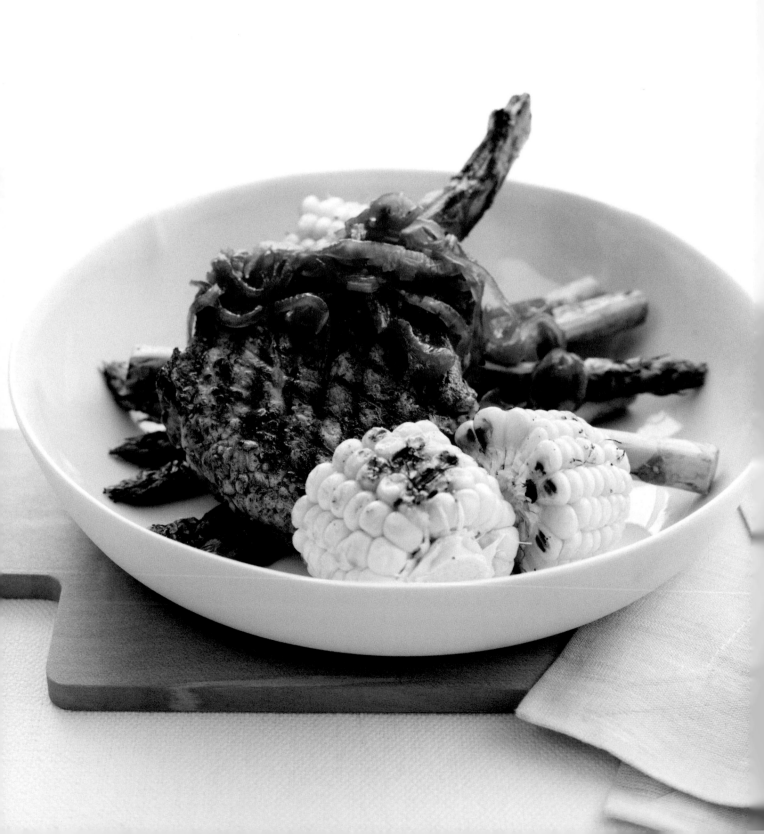

A dash of difference with seasonal vegetables cooked on the grill – bring out the sweetness and keep in the goodness.

veal cutlets with onion marmalade

PREPARATION TIME 15 MINUTES (PLUS REFRIGERATION TIME)
COOKING TIME 40 MINUTES **SERVES** 4

1 Combine oil, garlic and pepper in large bowl, add veal; toss veal to coat in marinade. Cover; refrigerate until required.
2 Meanwhile, heat butter in medium frying pan; cook onion, stirring, until soft and browned lightly. Add sugar, vinegar and juice; cook, stirring, about 15 minutes or until onion caramelises. Remove from heat; stir in rosemary.
3 Cook corn and asparagus, in batches, on heated oiled grill plate (or grill or barbecue) until browned lightly and cooked as desired; cover to keep warm.
4 Cook veal on same grill plate (or grill or barbecue) until cooked as desired. Serve veal, corn and asparagus topped with onion marmalade.

2 teaspoons olive oil

1 clove garlic, crushed

1 teaspoon cracked black pepper

4 veal cutlets (680g)

20g butter

2 large red onions (600g), sliced thinly

⅓ cup (75g) firmly packed brown sugar

¼ cup (60ml) apple cider vinegar

2 tablespoons orange juice

2 teaspoons finely chopped fresh rosemary

2 cobs corn (800g), trimmed, cut into 3cm pieces

500g asparagus, trimmed

NUTRITIONAL INFORMATION PER SERVING

11.7g total fat (4.1g saturated fat) **1965kJ (470 cal)** 50.8g carbohydrate **40.1g protein** 10.4g fibre

Baby squid hoods
are filled with fish
and served with salad
in this sensational,
simple summer meal.

squid stuffed with
smoked trout and basil

PREPARATION TIME 20 MINUTES **COOKING TIME** 10 MINUTES **SERVES** 4

1 small red onion (100g)

300g hot-smoked ocean trout
fillets, flaked coarsely

1 cup coarsely chopped fresh basil

8 baby squid hoods (500g), cleaned

100g baby rocket leaves

½ cup loosely packed fresh
flat-leaf parsley leaves

1 cup coarsely chopped fresh mint

¼ cup (60ml) white wine vinegar

1 tablespoon olive oil

2 limes, cut into 8 wedges

1 Slice half of the onion thinly; chop remaining half finely.
2 Combine chopped onion, fish and half of the basil in small bowl; fill hoods with fish mixture up to about 2cm from opening, secure with toothpicks.
3 Cook squid in heated lightly oiled large frying pan, uncovered, until browned lightly all over and tender.
4 Place rocket, parsley, mint, sliced onion and remaining basil in large bowl with combined vinegar and oil; toss gently to combine.
5 Cut squid in half on the diagonal; divide pieces among plates with salad and lime wedges.

NUTRITIONAL INFORMATION PER SERVING

10.3g total fat (2.1g saturated fat) **1158kJ (277 cal)** 2.6g carbohydrate **41.7g protein** 3g fibre

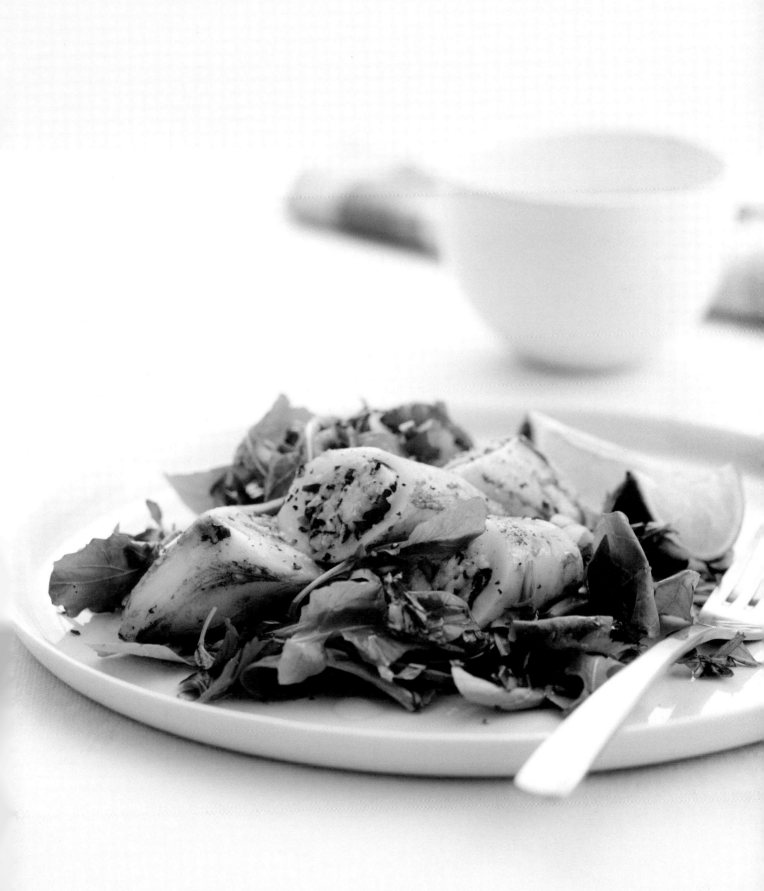

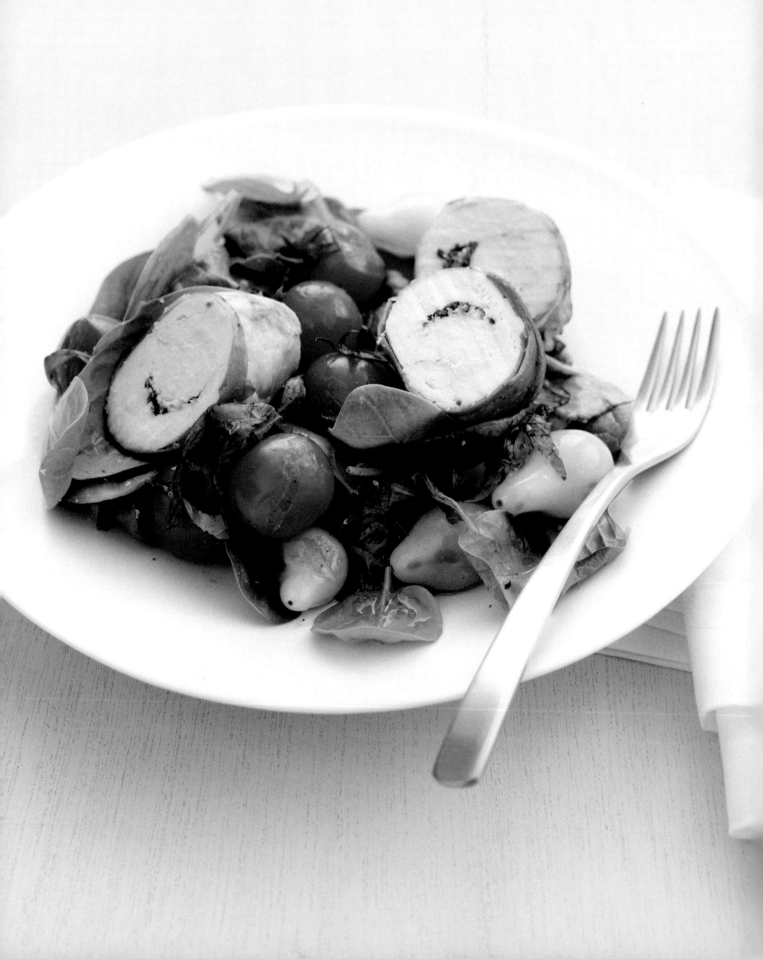

Pretty as a picture, these roll-ups can be cooked the day before, and served cold at a picnic.

herb-stuffed chicken with tomato salad

PREPARATION TIME 25 MINUTES **COOKING TIME** 25 MINUTES
SERVES 4

1 Preheat oven to moderate.
2 Combine finely chopped basil, oregano, thyme, garlic and rind in small bowl. Using meat mallet, gently pound chicken, one at a time, between pieces of plastic wrap until about 5mm thick. Divide herb mixture among chicken pieces; roll to enclose filling, wrapping each roll with prosciutto slice to secure.
3 Cook chicken in heated lightly oiled large frying pan, uncovered, about 10 minutes or until browned all over. Place chicken on oven tray; cook, uncovered, in moderate oven about 15 minutes or until cooked through.
4 Meanwhile, cook tomatoes in same pan, over high heat, stirring, 3 minutes. Gently toss tomatoes, spinach and coarsely chopped basil in large bowl with combined vinegar and oil. Serve salad with chicken.

¼ cup finely chopped fresh basil

1 tablespoon finely chopped fresh oregano

2 teaspoons fresh lemon thyme

2 cloves garlic, crushed

1 tablespoon finely grated lemon rind

4 single chicken breast fillets (680g)

4 slices prosciutto (60g)

250g cherry tomatoes

250g teardrop tomatoes

150g baby spinach leaves

½ cup coarsely chopped fresh basil

2 tablespoons red wine vinegar

2 teaspoons olive oil

NUTRITIONAL INFORMATION PER SERVING

7.4g total fat (1.7g saturated fat) **1066kJ (255 cal)** 3.4g carbohydrate **42.9g protein** 3.6g fibre

Use the large shells to
scoop up mouthfuls
of spicy juices.

thai-flavoured mussels

PREPARATION TIME 30 MINUTES **COOKING TIME** 10 MINUTES **SERVES** 4

*When removing the leaves from a bunch of coriander, remove
some of the stems and roots for this recipe.*

2kg large black mussels

2 tablespoons water

⅓ cup (80ml) lime juice

2 tablespoons grated palm sugar

2 tablespoons fish sauce

1 fresh long red chilli,
chopped finely

2 teaspoons peanut oil

10cm stick (20g) finely chopped
fresh lemon grass

1 clove garlic, crushed

4cm piece fresh ginger (20g), grated

2 teaspoons finely chopped
coriander roots and stems

2 green onions, sliced thinly

½ cup firmly packed fresh
coriander leaves

½ cup firmly packed fresh
thai basil leaves

2 fresh long red chillies,
sliced thinly

1 Scrub mussels under cold water; discard beards.
2 Whisk the water, juice, sugar, sauce and chopped chilli in small jug.
3 Heat oil in large saucepan; cook lemon grass, garlic, ginger and coriander roots and stems, stirring, until fragrant. Stir in lime mixture; bring to a boil. Add mussels; return to a boil. Reduce heat; simmer, covered, about 5 minutes or until mussels open (discard any that do not).
4 Divide mussels and cooking liquid among plates; sprinkle with onion, coriander leaves, basil and sliced chilli.

NUTRITIONAL INFORMATION PER SERVING

4.2g total fat (0.9g saturated fat) **594kJ (142 cal)** 12.5g carbohydrate **13.1g protein** 0.9g fibre

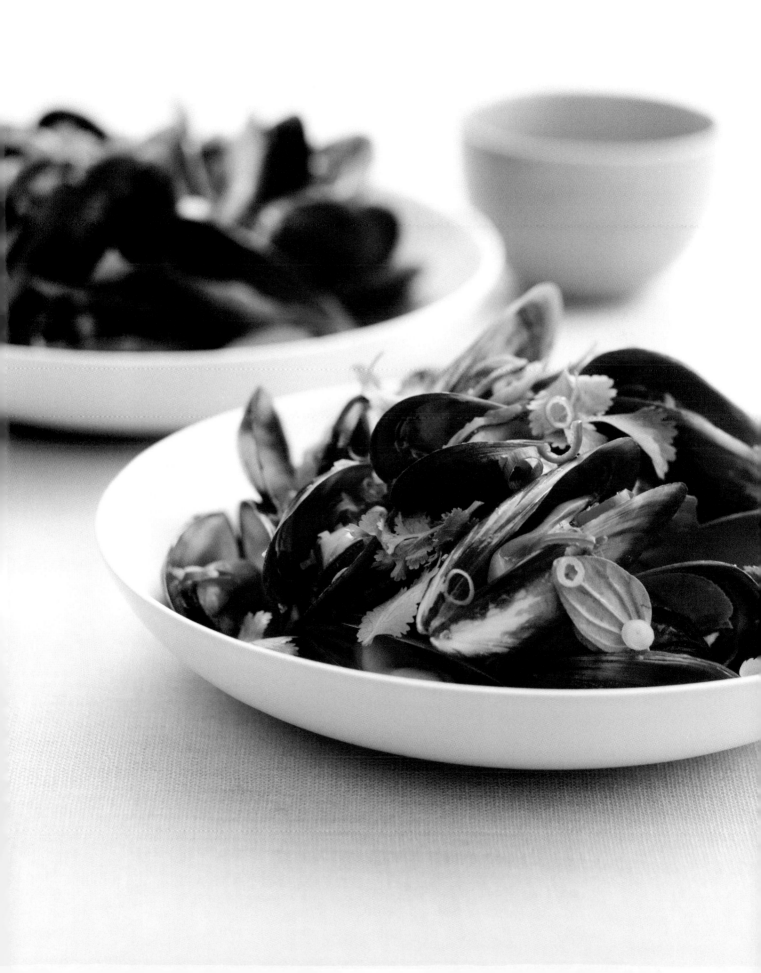

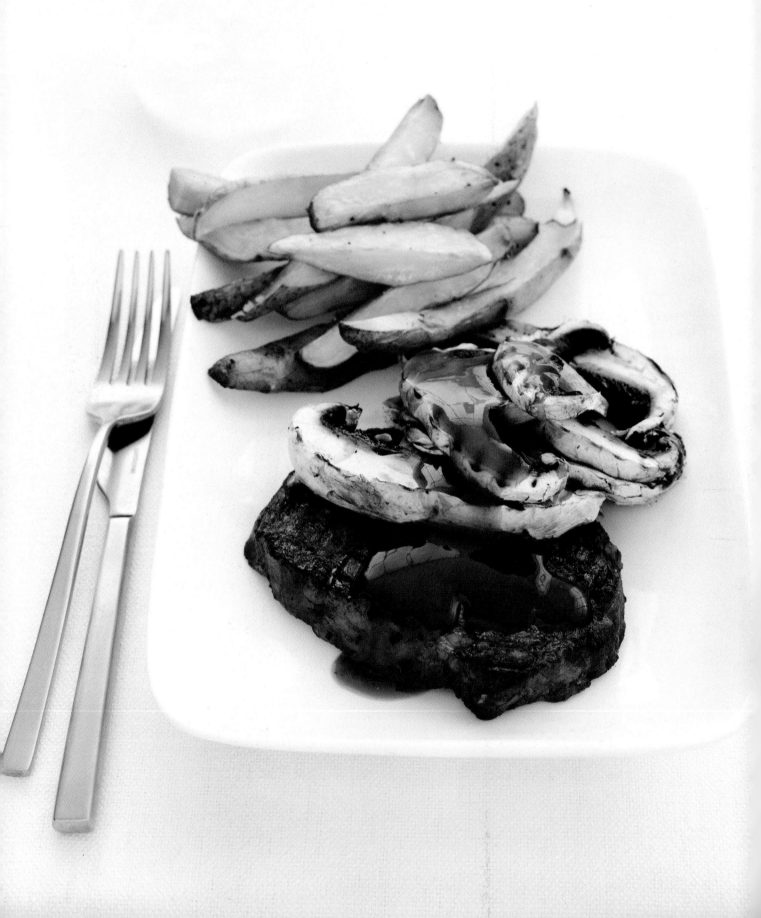

Meat and potatoes
done up to dazzle.

balsamic-seared steak with kipflers and mushrooms

PREPARATION TIME 15 MINUTES (PLUS REFRIGERATION TIME)
COOKING TIME 15 MINUTES **SERVES** 4

1 Combine vinegar and garlic in medium bowl, add beef; toss beef to coat in marinade. Cover; refrigerate 3 hours or overnight.
2 Preheat oven to moderately hot.
3 Place potato, in single layer, in large shallow baking dish; drizzle with oil. Roast, uncovered, in moderately hot oven, stirring occasionally, about 30 minutes or until browned lightly and crisp.
4 Meanwhile, cook steaks on heated lightly oiled grill plate (or grill or barbecue) until cooked as desired. Cover to keep warm.
5 Cook mushroom on same heated grill plate (or grill or barbecue) until just tender.
6 Place wine in small saucepan; bring to a boil. Add jam and blended cornflour and stock; stir until sauce boils and thickens slightly. Serve steaks with mushrooms, potato and sauce.

¼ cup (60ml) balsamic vinegar

2 cloves garlic, crushed

4 beef scotch fillet steaks (800g)

1kg kipfler potatoes, quartered lengthways

1 tablespoon olive oil

500g flat mushrooms, sliced thickly

2 tablespoons dry red wine

1 tablespoon plum jam

1 tablespoon cornflour

¾ cup (180ml) beef stock

NUTRITIONAL INFORMATION PER SERVING

13.7g total fat (4.3g saturated fat) **2165kJ (518 cal)** 40.8g carbohydrate **54.2g protein** 8.4g fibre

Sumac struts its stuff on this stage, bringing a mysterious quality that is slightly sour, faintly fruity, and purple-red in hue.

sumac, salt and pepper fish with mediterranean salad

PREPARATION TIME 20 MINUTES **COOKING TIME** 10 MINUTES **SERVES** 4

We used blue-eye for this recipe, but you can use any firm white-fleshed fish fillets.

2 tablespoons sumac

1 teaspoon salt

1 teaspoon cracked black pepper

4 blue-eye fillets (800g)

1 cup (200g) couscous

1 cup (250ml) boiling water

1 tablespoon olive oil

1 lemon, quartered

MEDITERRANEAN SALAD

2 medium tomatoes (300g), seeded, chopped coarsely

2 medium red capsicums (400g), chopped coarsely

2 tablespoons seeded kalamata olives, chopped coarsely

2 tablespoons drained baby capers, rinsed

1 cup coarsely chopped fresh flat-leaf parsley

1 Combine sumac, salt and pepper in large bowl, add fish; turn fish to coat in mixture. Cook fish, in batches, in heated lightly oiled large frying pan until cooked as desired.

2 Meanwhile, place mediterranean salad ingredients in medium bowl; toss gently to combine.

3 Combine couscous with the water in large heatproof bowl. Cover; stand about 5 minutes or until water is absorbed, fluffing with fork occasionally. Stir in oil.

4 Divide couscous among plates, top with salad and fish; serve with lemon.

NUTRITIONAL INFORMATION PER SERVING

9.7g total fat (2.1g saturated fat) **1990kJ (476 cal)** 45.7g carbohydrate **49.9g protein** 3.9g fibre

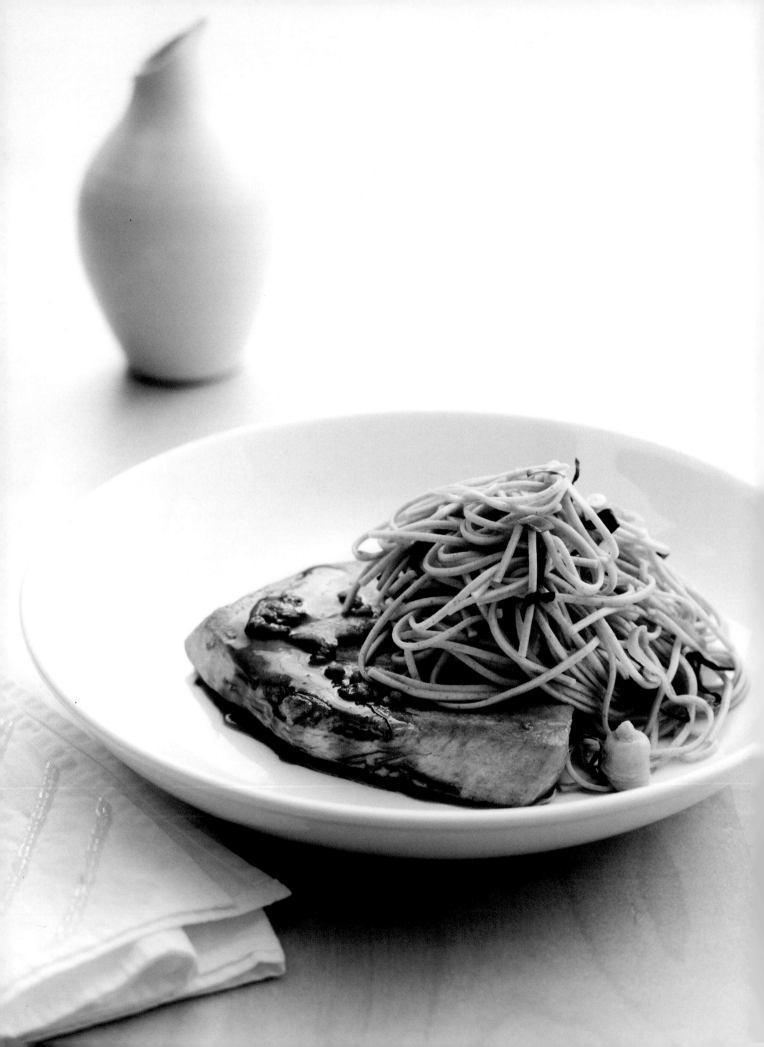

Sake, soba and
seaweed make this
a tribute to Japan.

seared tuna
with chilled soba

PREPARATION TIME 15 MINUTES (PLUS REFRIGERATION TIME)
COOKING TIME 5 MINUTES **SERVES** 4

1 Cook soba in large saucepan of boiling water, uncovered, until just tender; drain. Rinse under cold water; drain. Place in medium bowl, cover; refrigerate until required.
2 Meanwhile, combine mirin, kecap manis, sake, sugar, fresh ginger and garlic in small jug.
3 Cook fish in heated lightly oiled large frying pan, uncovered, until cooked as desired (tuna can become very dry if overcooked; we recommend you sear it over very high heat for about 30 seconds each side). Add mirin mixture to pan; coat fish both sides in mixture. Remove fish from pan; cover to keep warm.
4 Bring mixture in pan to a boil. Reduce heat; simmer, uncovered, 30 seconds. Strain sauce into small jug.
5 Meanwhile, place seaweed, onion, oil and pickled ginger in bowl with soba; toss gently to combine. Divide fish among plates, drizzle with sauce; top with soba. Serve with wasabi, if desired.

200g dried soba

¼ cup (60ml) mirin

2 tablespoons kecap manis

1 tablespoon cooking sake

2 teaspoons white sugar

5cm piece fresh ginger (25g), grated

1 clove garlic, crushed

4 tuna steaks (800g)

1 sheet toasted seaweed (yaki-nori), sliced thinly

2 green onions, chopped finely

1 teaspoon sesame oil

2 tablespoons pickled ginger, sliced thinly

NUTRITIONAL INFORMATION PER SERVING

13.2g total fat (4.9g saturated fat) **2182kJ (522 cal)** 41.9g carbohydrate **56.3g protein** 2.6g fibre

East meets mex in
a hip wrap you can
eat on the hop.

glazed-chicken tortilla with sprout and herb salad

PREPARATION TIME 15 MINUTES **COOKING TIME** 20 MINUTES **SERVES** 4

¼ cup (80g) cranberry sauce

1 tablespoon wholegrain mustard

1 tablespoon lemon juice

5cm piece fresh ginger (25g), grated

1 clove garlic, crushed

500g chicken breast fillets

1 small red onion (100g),
sliced thinly

60g snow pea sprouts

¼ cup thinly sliced fresh coriander

¼ cup thinly sliced fresh mint

1 tablespoon white wine vinegar

4 large flour tortillas

1 Heat combined sauce, mustard, juice, ginger and garlic in small saucepan, stirring, until glaze comes to a boil.
2 Cook chicken, in batches, in heated lightly oiled large frying pan, brushing frequently with glaze, until cooked through. Cover chicken; stand 5 minutes before slicing thickly.
3 Meanwhile, place onion, sprouts, herbs and vinegar in medium bowl; toss salad gently to combine. Heat tortillas according to manufacturer's instructions.
4 Divide chicken and salad among centres of tortillas; roll tortillas around filling to form cone shapes.

NUTRITIONAL INFORMATION PER SERVING

5.6g total fat (1.2g saturated fat) **1296kJ (310 cal)** 31g carbohydrate **33.4g protein** 2.9g fibre

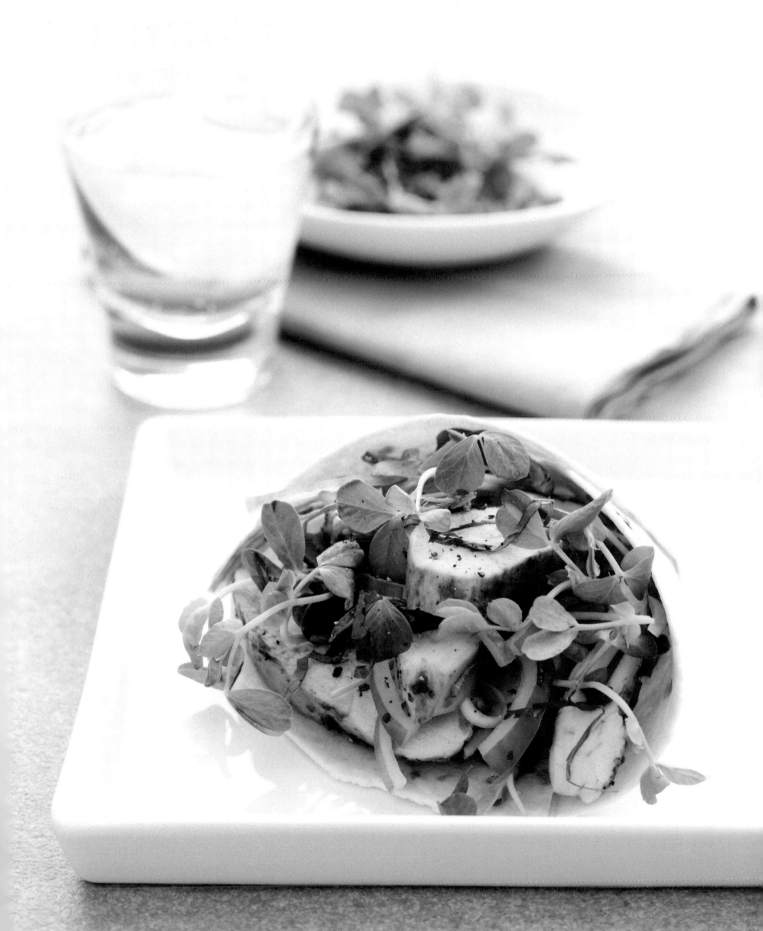

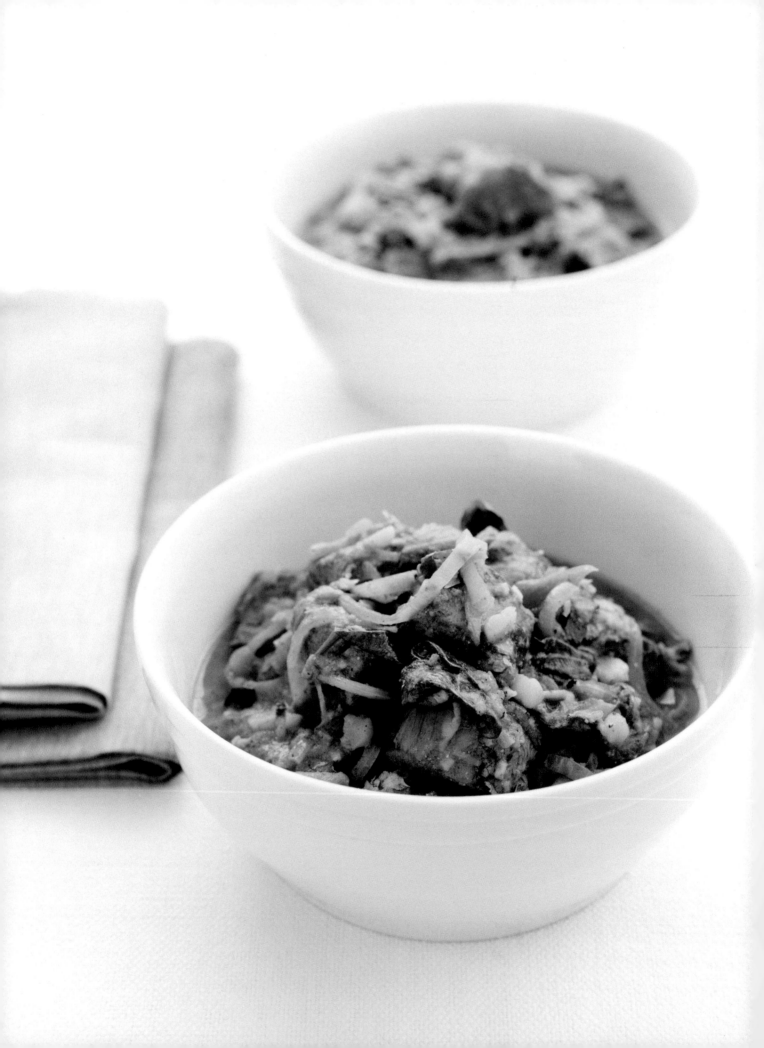

Sweet and pungent
spices create flavour.

lamb and lentil curry

PREPARATION TIME 15 MINUTES **COOKING TIME** 55 MINUTES
SERVES 4

1 Cook split peas in medium saucepan of boiling water, uncovered, until just tender; drain.
2 Meanwhile, heat half of the oil in large saucepan; cook lamb, in batches, stirring, until cooked as desired. Drain on absorbent paper.
3 Heat remaining oil in same pan; cook onion, stirring, about 15 minutes or until caramelised. Add ginger, garlic, ground coriander, paprika and cayenne; cook, stirring, until fragrant. Add yogurt; cook 5 minutes, without boiling, stirring occasionally.
4 Add tomato, stock and coconut cream; bring to a boil. Reduce heat; simmer, uncovered, about 15 minutes or until sauce thickens slightly.
5 Return lamb to pan with split peas and spinach; cook, stirring, until heated through. Remove from heat; stir in fresh coriander.

1 cup (200g) yellow split peas

1 tablespoon olive oil

600g lamb fillets, diced into 4cm pieces

2 large brown onions (400g), sliced thinly

5cm piece fresh ginger (25g), chopped finely

2 cloves garlic, crushed

2 tablespoons ground coriander

1 tablespoon sweet paprika

½ teaspoon cayenne pepper

200g yogurt

2 medium tomatoes (300g), chopped coarsely

1¾ cups (430ml) chicken stock

⅔ cup (160ml) light coconut cream

150g baby spinach leaves

⅓ cup coarsely chopped fresh coriander

NUTRITIONAL INFORMATION PER SERVING

19.3g total fat (9.8g saturated fat) **2153kJ (515 cal)** 33.5g carbohydrate **51.7g protein** 8.9g fibre

grilled lamb cutlets
with warm risoni salad

PREPARATION TIME 15 MINUTES (PLUS REFRIGERATION TIME)
COOKING TIME 35 MINUTES **SERVES** 4

*Risoni is a small rice-shaped pasta very similar to orzo;
you can use either for this recipe.*

1 clove garlic, crushed

1 tablespoon finely chopped
fresh oregano

1 tablespoon finely chopped
fresh chives

2 tablespoons lemon juice

¼ cup (60ml) dry white wine

12 french-trimmed lamb
cutlets (700g)

WARM RISONI SALAD

500g pumpkin, diced into
3cm pieces

1 clove garlic, crushed

1 tablespoon olive oil

1 cup (220g) risoni

150g baby spinach leaves

2 tablespoons lemon juice

2 tablespoons coarsely chopped
fresh chives

2 tablespoons fresh oregano leaves

1 Combine garlic, oregano, chives, juice and wine in large bowl, add
   lamb; toss lamb to coat in marinade. Cover; refrigerate until required.
2 Meanwhile, make warm risoni salad.
3 Drain lamb; discard marinade. Cook lamb, in batches, on heated
   lightly oiled grill plate (or grill or barbecue) until cooked as desired.
   Serve cutlets with salad.

WARM RISONI SALAD Preheat oven to moderately hot. Place pumpkin,
in single layer, on oven tray; drizzle with combined garlic and half of
the oil. Roast, uncovered, in moderately hot oven about 15 minutes
or until pumpkin is browned lightly and tender. Meanwhile, cook pasta
in large saucepan of boiling water, uncovered, until just tender; drain.
Combine pasta and spinach in large bowl with pumpkin, juice, herbs
and remaining oil; toss gently to combine.

NUTRITIONAL INFORMATION PER SERVING

11.5g total fat (3.6g saturated fat) **1735kJ (415 cal)** 46.4g carbohydrate **28g protein** 5.4g fibre

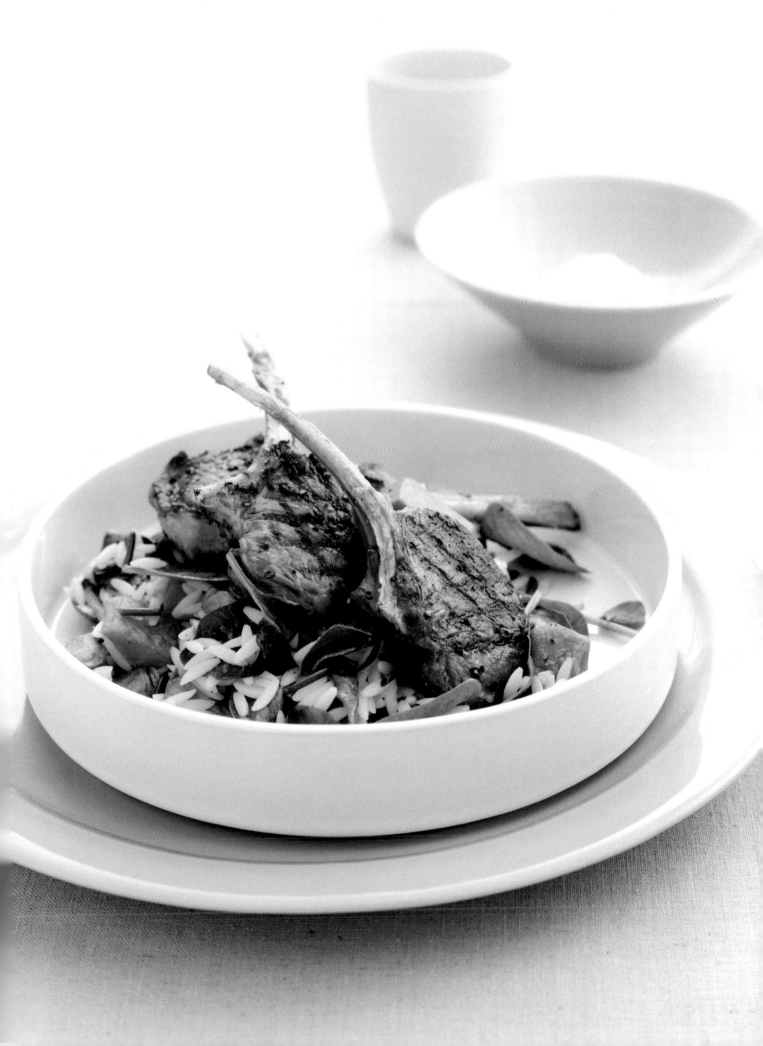

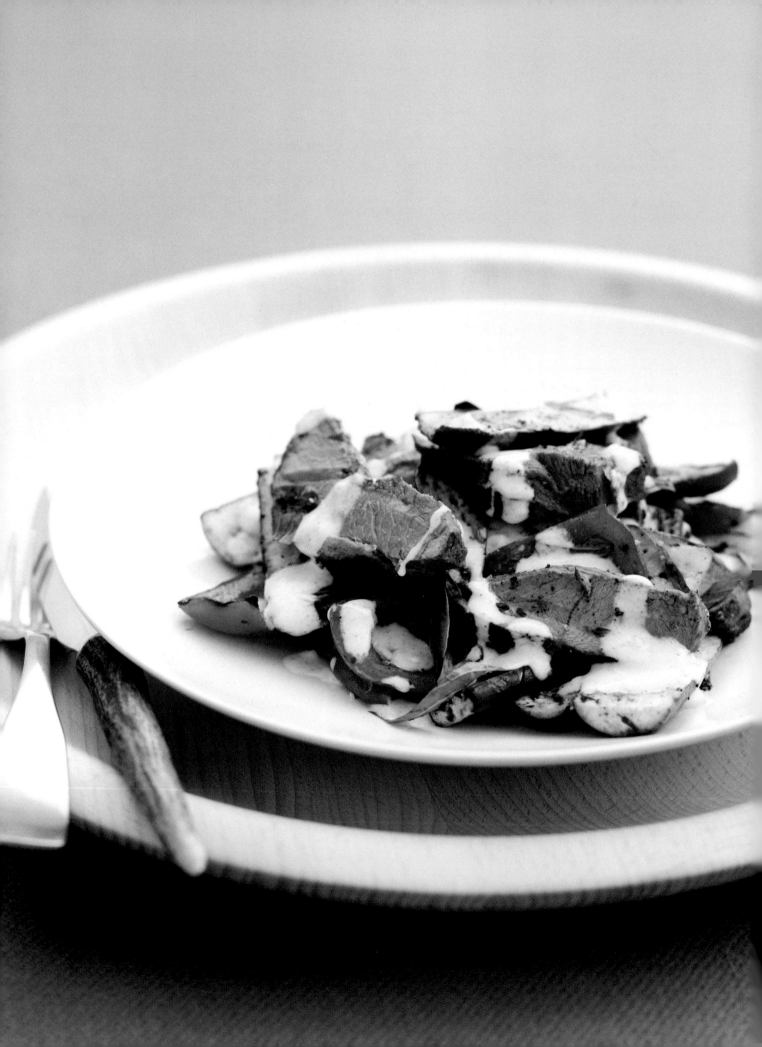

harissa-scented lamb with char-grilled vegetables

PREPARATION TIME 20 MINUTES **COOKING TIME** 30 MINUTES **SERVES** 6

Harissa, a Moroccan sauce or paste made from dried red chillies, garlic oil and caraway seeds, can be used as a rub for meat, an ingredient in sauces and dressings, or eaten on its own as a condiment. It is available commercially from supermarkets.

Shake it up baby for a dazzling garlic sauce that brings together this exotic lamb dish.

1 Combine garlic sauce ingredients in screw-top jar; shake well.
2 Combine crushed garlic, rind, harissa and half of the juice in large bowl, add lamb; toss lamb to coat in mixture.
3 Cook lamb on heated lightly oiled grill plate (or grill or barbecue), covered, about 20 minutes or until lamb is cooked as desired. Cover lamb; stand 5 minutes before slicing thickly.
4 Meanwhile, combine capsicum, zucchini, eggplant, cumin and remaining juice in large bowl. Cook vegetables on same grill plate (or grill or barbecue) until just tender. Return vegetables to bowl with herbs; toss gently to combine.
5 Serve lamb with char-grilled vegetables; drizzle with garlic sauce.

3 cloves garlic, crushed

1 tablespoon finely grated lemon rind

2 tablespoons harissa

1/3 cup (80ml) lemon juice

1.5kg butterflied leg of lamb, trimmed

2 medium red capsicums (400g), sliced thickly

3 large zucchini (450g), sliced thickly

8 baby eggplants (480g), sliced thickly

1 teaspoon ground cumin

1 tablespoon fresh thyme leaves

1/2 cup coarsely chopped fresh mint

GARLIC SAUCE

1 clove garlic, crushed

1 teaspoon ground cumin

1/2 cup (125ml) buttermilk

1/3 cup (95g) low-fat yogurt

NUTRITIONAL INFORMATION PER SERVING

7g total fat (3g saturated fat) **1780kJ (354 cal)** 9.7g carbohydrate **61.6g protein** 4.3g fibre

pepper-crusted beef fillet with vegetable and polenta chips

PREPARATION TIME 20 MINUTES (PLUS REFRIGERATION TIME)
COOKING TIME 1 HOUR 5 MINUTES **SERVES** 4

3 cups (750ml) water

¾ cup (120g) polenta

2 tablespoons wholegrain mustard

2 teaspoons cracked black pepper

600g beef eye fillet

1 large kumara (500g)

2 large parsnips (700g)

2 large carrots (360g)

2 teaspoons olive oil

cooking-oil spray

½ cup coarsely chopped fresh flat-leaf parsley

¼ cup (60ml) balsamic vinegar

¼ cup (60ml) water, extra

1 tablespoon wholegrain mustard, extra

1 tablespoon honey

1 Lightly oil deep 23cm-square cake pan.

2 Bring the water to a boil in medium saucepan. Gradually add polenta to liquid, stirring constantly. Reduce heat; cook, stirring constantly, about 10 minutes or until polenta thickens. Stir in half of the mustard; spread polenta into prepared pan. Cover; refrigerate about 1 hour or until firm.

3 Preheat oven to moderately hot.

4 Spread combined remaining mustard and pepper all over beef. Cut peeled vegetables into similar-sized baton shapes. Place combined vegetables, in single layer, in large shallow flameproof baking dish; drizzle with oil. Roast, uncovered, in moderately hot oven 10 minutes. Add beef to dish; roast, uncovered, in moderately hot oven about 35 minutes or until vegetables are crisp and beef is cooked as desired.

5 Meanwhile, turn polenta onto board; cut into baton shapes similar to vegetables. Coat polenta with cooking-oil spray; place, in single layer, on oven tray. Place polenta in same oven with beef and vegetables for about the last 20 minutes of cooking time or until browned lightly.

6 Remove beef from baking dish. Cover beef; stand 5 minutes before slicing thinly. Place vegetables in large bowl with parsley; toss gently to combine. Cover to keep warm.

7 Place baking dish over high heat; add vinegar, the extra water, extra mustard and honey. Cook, stirring, about 5 minutes or until sauce bubbles and thickens.

8 Serve vegetables, polenta and beef, drizzled with sauce.

NUTRITIONAL INFORMATION PER SERVING

11.1g total fat (3.3g saturated fat) **2140kJ (512 cal)** 61.1g carbohydrate **40.7g protein** 9.6g fibre

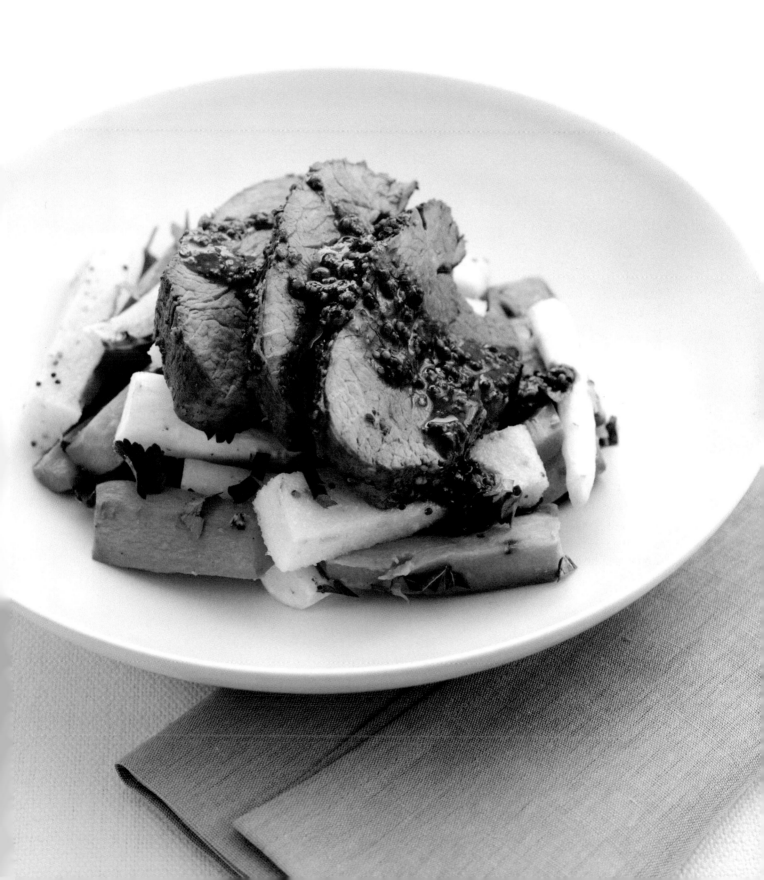

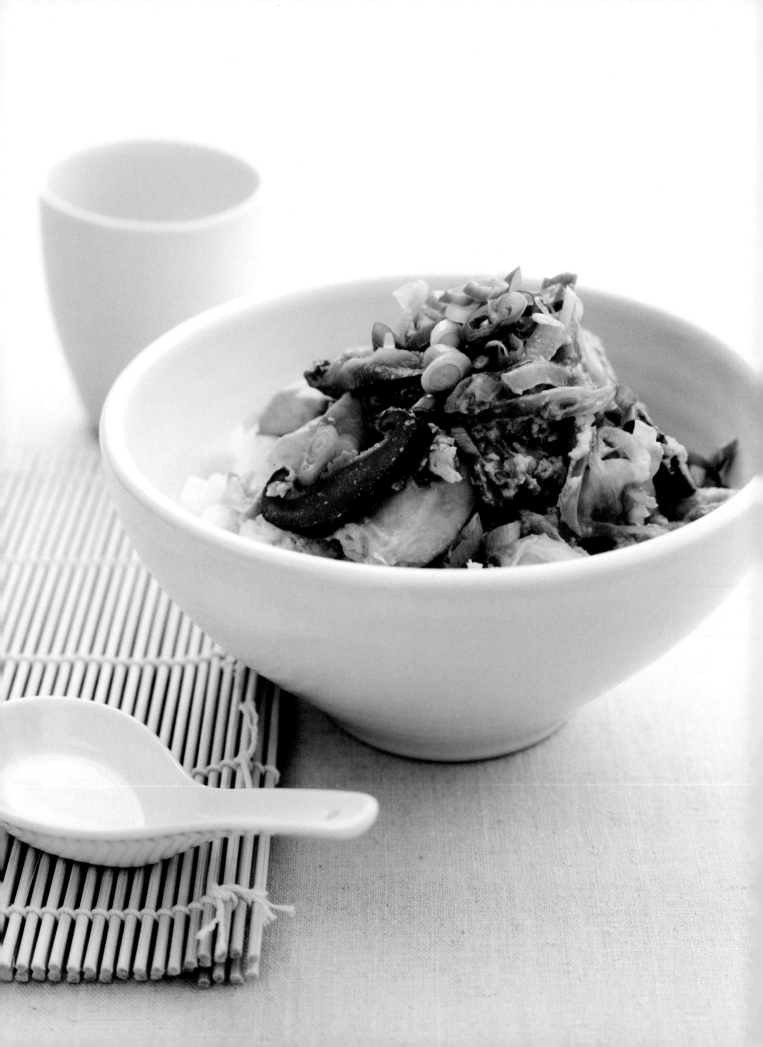

chicken donburi

PREPARATION TIME 20 MINUTES (PLUS STANDING TIME)
COOKING TIME 40 MINUTES **SERVES** 4

*A Japanese culinary term, donburi is made with rice,
vegetables and a single variety of any meat; it is also
the name given to the dish in which this recipe is cooked.
This version, oyako donburi, translates as parent and child,
as it's made with both chicken and eggs.*

1 Place mushrooms in small heatproof bowl, cover with boiling water, stand 20 minutes; drain. Discard stems; slice caps thinly.
2 Meanwhile, combine dashi with the boiling water in small jug.
3 Cook brown onion in heated lightly oiled large frying pan, stirring, about 10 minutes or until onion is browned lightly. Add half of the dashi mixture, reduce heat; simmer, stirring occasionally, about 10 minutes or until softened. Transfer to medium bowl.
4 Bring rice and the cold water to a boil in large saucepan, uncovered, stirring occasionally. Reduce heat to as low as possible; cover with a tight-fitting lid, cook rice 12 minutes. Do not remove lid or stir rice during cooking time. Remove from heat; stand, covered, 10 minutes.
5 Meanwhile, combine remaining dashi mixture with sauce, mirin and sugar in same frying pan; bring to a boil. Add chicken and mushroom; cook, covered, about 5 minutes or until chicken is cooked through.
6 Combine egg with cooked onion in bowl, pour over chicken mixture; cook, covered, over low heat, about 5 minutes or until egg just sets.
7 Divide rice among serving bowls; top with chicken mixture, sprinkle with green onion.

4 dried shiitake mushrooms

½ teaspoon dashi powder

1 cup (250ml) boiling water

4 medium brown onions (600g), sliced thinly

1½ cups (300g) koshihikari rice

3 cups (750ml) cold water

¼ cup (60ml) soy sauce

2 tablespoons mirin

1 teaspoon white sugar

600g chicken breast fillets, chopped coarsely

4 eggs, beaten lightly

2 green onions, sliced thinly

NUTRITIONAL INFORMATION PER SERVING

9.4g total fat (2.7g saturated fat) **2328kJ (557 cal)** 67.9g carbohydrate **48.9g protein** 2.9g fibre

DESSERTS

Every cook needs
a one-size-fits-all
dessert – something
light, easy, reliable,
and delicious enough
to complement any
meal and a busy life.

brown-sugar meringues with banana and caramel sauce

PREPARATION TIME 15 MINUTES **COOKING TIME** 1 HOUR **SERVES** 4

3 egg whites

¾ cup (165g) firmly packed
dark brown sugar

3 teaspoons cornflour

3 teaspoons white vinegar

1 teaspoon vanilla extract

10g butter

⅓ cup (80ml) light cream

¼ cup (55g) firmly packed
dark brown sugar, extra

2 medium bananas (400g),
sliced thinly

1 Preheat oven to very slow.
2 Beat egg whites in small bowl with electric mixer until soft peaks
   form. Gradually add sugar, 1 tablespoon at a time, beating until
   sugar dissolves between additions; fold in cornflour, vinegar
   and extract.
3 Divide meringue mixture among four shallow ¾-cup (180ml) ovenproof
   dishes. Place dishes on oven tray; bake, uncovered, in very slow
   oven about 1 hour or until meringues are firm.
4 Meanwhile, melt butter in small saucepan, add cream and extra
   sugar; bring to a boil. Reduce heat; simmer, uncovered, about
   2 minutes or until mixture thickens slightly.
5 Divide banana slices among meringues; drizzle with caramel sauce.

NUTRITIONAL INFORMATION PER SERVING

7.5g total fat (4.9g saturated fat) **1463kJ (350 cal)** 69.1g carbohydrate **4.5g protein** 1.5g fibre

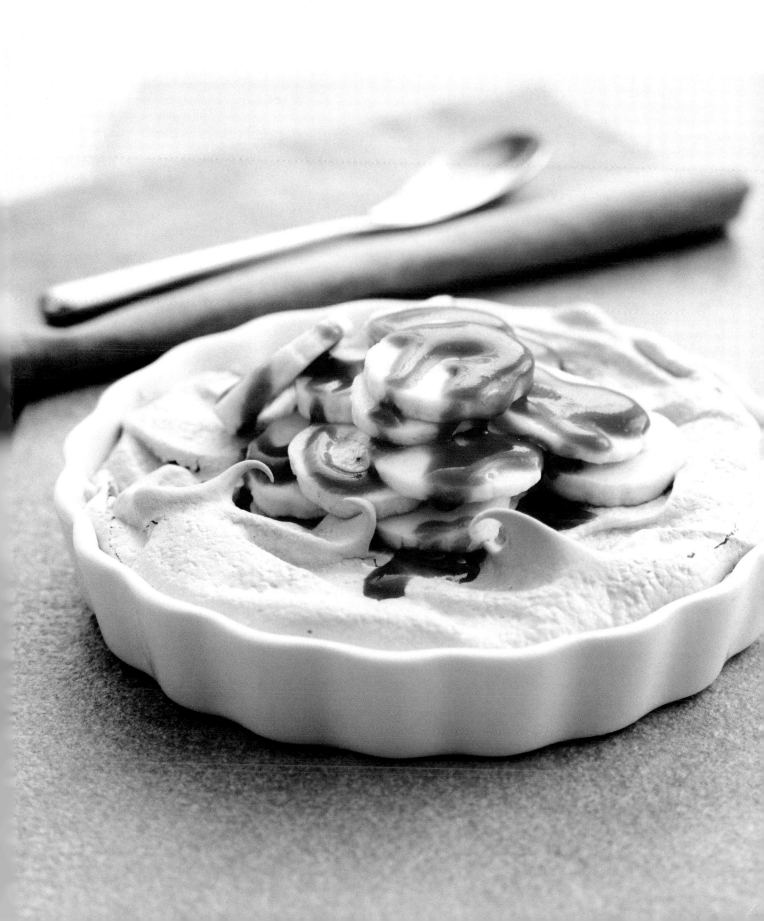

frozen passionfruit yogurt

PREPARATION TIME 10 MINUTES (PLUS FREEZING TIME)   COOKING TIME 5 MINUTES   SERVES 4

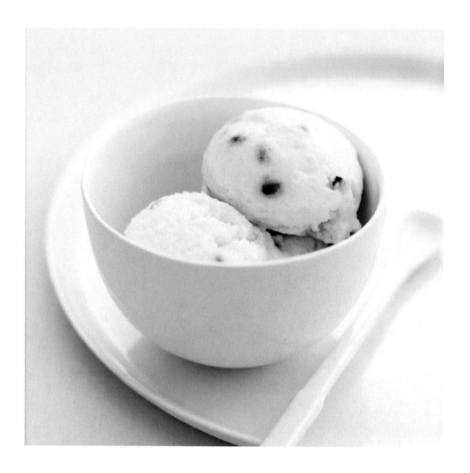

½ cup (110g) caster sugar

¼ cup (60ml) water

1 teaspoon gelatine

2 cups (560g) low-fat yogurt

½ cup (125ml) passionfruit pulp

You need approximately six passionfruit for this recipe.

1 Combine sugar and the water in small saucepan, stirring over low heat until sugar dissolves; transfer to medium jug.
2 Sprinkle gelatine over sugar syrup, stirring until gelatine dissolves.
3 Combine yogurt and pulp in jug with syrup. Pour yogurt mixture into loaf pan, cover tightly with foil; freeze 3 hours or until almost set. Scrape yogurt from bottom and sides of pan with fork; return to freezer until firm.

NUTRITIONAL INFORMATION PER SERVING

2.5g total fat (1.5g saturated fat) **924kJ (221 cal)** 39.9g carbohydrate **8.6g protein** 4.3g fibre

caramelised figs with spiced yogurt

PREPARATION TIME 10 MINUTES **COOKING TIME** 10 MINUTES **SERVES** 4

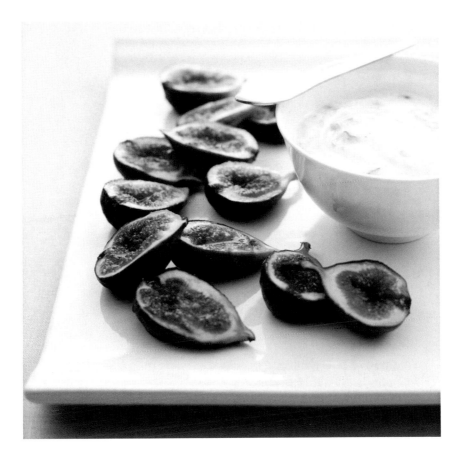

1 Combine yogurt, nuts, nutmeg and sugar in small bowl.
2 Halve figs lengthways. Brush cut-side of figs with honey.
3 Cook figs, cut-side down, uncovered, in heated large non-stick frying pan 5 minutes. Turn figs; cook, uncovered, 5 minutes or until browned lightly. Serve figs with spiced yogurt.

1 cup (280g) low-fat yogurt

¼ cup (35g) toasted pistachios, chopped coarsely

¼ teaspoon ground nutmeg

1 tablespoon caster sugar

6 large fresh figs (480g)

1 tablespoon honey

NUTRITIONAL INFORMATION PER SERVING

6g total fat (1.3g saturated fat) **777kJ (186 cal)** 26.1g carbohydrate **6.8g protein** 3.6g fibre

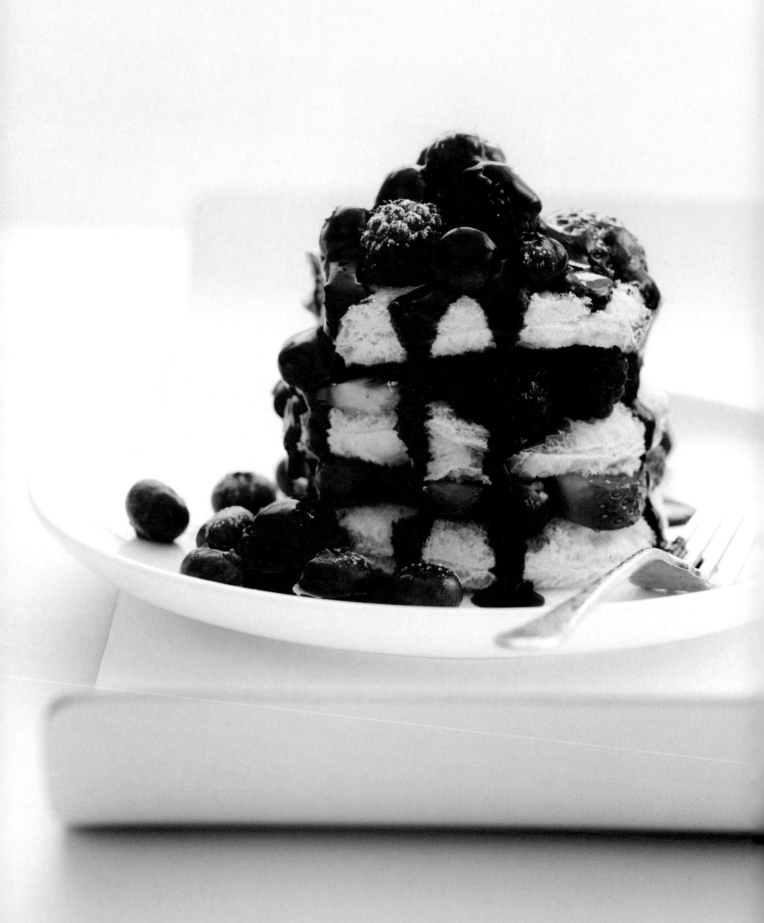

The height of
sophistication, this is
superb to serve when
the weather is warm.

summer berry stack

PREPARATION TIME 20 MINUTES **COOKING TIME** 5 MINUTES
SERVES 4

1 Make blackberry coulis.
2 Cut twelve 1cm-thick slices from brioche loaf; using 7cm cutter, cut one round from each slice.
3 Combine berries in medium bowl.
4 Place one round on each plate; divide a third of the berries among rounds. Place another round on top of each stack; divide half of the remaining berries among stacks. Place remaining rounds on berry stacks; top with remaining berries.
5 Pour coulis over stacks; dust each with sifted icing sugar.

BLACKBERRY COULIS Stir ingredients in medium saucepan over high heat; bring to a boil. Reduce heat; simmer, uncovered, 3 minutes. Strain coulis into medium jug; cool 10 minutes.

TIP Toast any leftover brioche loaf for breakfast, or use it to make a bread and butter pudding.

450g brioche loaf

250g strawberries, sliced thickly

150g raspberries

150g blueberries

1 tablespoon icing sugar mixture

BLACKBERRY COULIS

300g frozen blackberries

¼ cup (40g) icing sugar mixture

¼ cup (60ml) water

NUTRITIONAL INFORMATION PER SERVING

7.2g total fat (3g saturated fat) **1313kJ (314 cal)** 55.3g carbohydrate **7.5g protein** 9.7g fibre

tropical fruit sorbets

PREPARATION TIME 20 MINUTES (PLUS FREEZING TIME)
COOKING TIME 10 MINUTES **SERVES** 4

The basic sorbet mixture makes four servings; use only one of the three different fruit flavours given below for that amount of sorbet. However, if you wish, you can make all three flavours by tripling the basic sorbet recipe.

½ cup (125ml) water
½ cup (110g) caster sugar
2 egg whites

1 Stir the water and sugar in small saucepan over heat until sugar dissolves; bring to a boil. Reduce heat; simmer, uncovered, without stirring, 5 minutes. Transfer to large heatproof jug, cool 10 minutes.
2 Meanwhile, blend or process fruit of your choice (see recipes below) until pureed. You need 2 cups of fruit puree for this recipe; freeze any that is left over. Stir puree into sugar syrup.
3 Pour sorbet mixture into loaf pan, cover tightly with foil; freeze 3 hours or overnight.
4 Blend or process mixture with egg whites until smooth. Return to loaf pan, cover; freeze until firm.

PINEAPPLE Blend or process 1 small peeled and coarsely chopped pineapple (900g) then follow the basic sorbet recipe in Step 2 above.

NUTRITIONAL INFORMATION PER SERVING

0.1g total fat (0g saturated fat) **656kJ (157 cal)**
36.9g carbohydrate **3g protein** 2.5g fibre

KIWIFRUIT Blend or process 7 medium peeled kiwifruit (600g) then follow the basic sorbet recipe in Step 2 above.

NUTRITIONAL INFORMATION PER SERVING

0.3g total fat (0g saturated fat) **732kJ (175 cal)** 40.1g carbohydrate **3.6g protein** 4.2g fibre

MANGO Blend or process 3 small peeled and seeded mangoes (900g) then follow the basic sorbet recipe in Step 2 above.

NUTRITIONAL INFORMATION PER SERVING

0.3g total fat (0g saturated fat) **849kJ (203 cal)** 47.7g carbohydrate **3.4g protein** 2.4g fibre

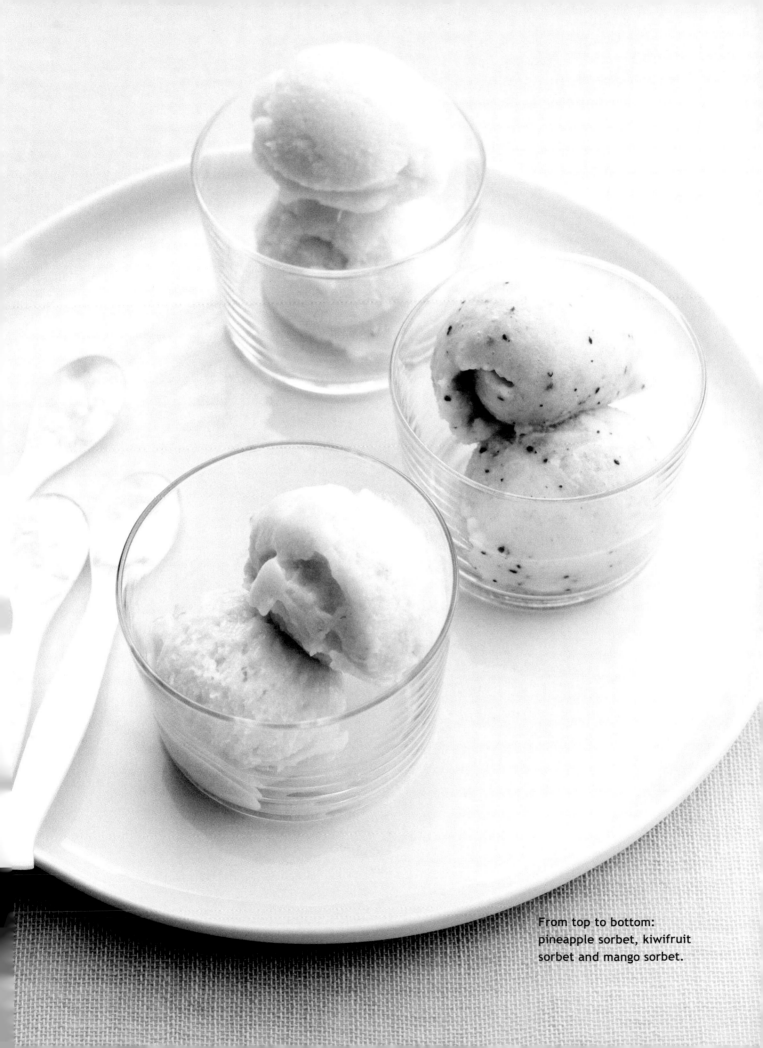

From top to bottom:
pineapple sorbet, kiwifruit
sorbet and mango sorbet.

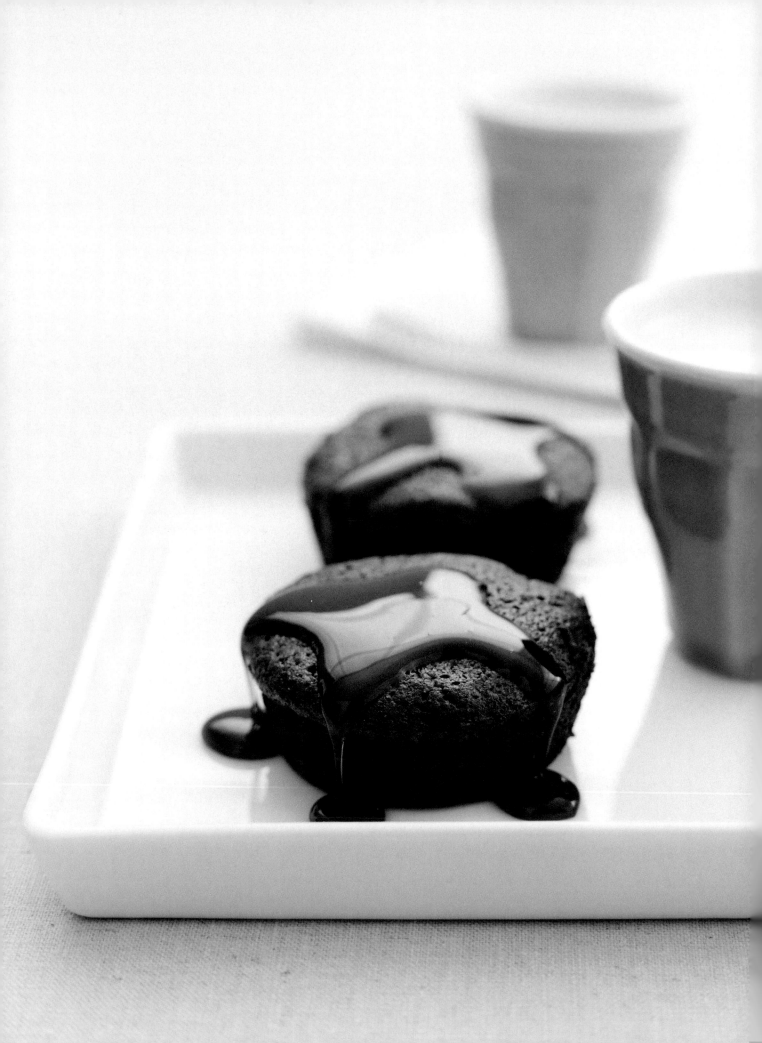

Turn a classic choc indulgence into a mocha masterpiece.

chocolate fudge cakes with coffee syrup

PREPARATION TIME 15 MINUTES **COOKING TIME** 20 MINUTES
MAKES 12

1 Preheat oven to moderately slow. Lightly grease 12-hole (⅓-cup/80ml) muffin pan.
2 Combine sifted cocoa and sugar in large bowl; blend in the water then chocolate, stir until smooth. Stir in egg yolks, almond meal and flour.
3 Beat egg whites in small bowl with electric mixer until soft peaks form. Fold egg whites into chocolate mixture, in two batches; divide mixture among prepared holes of muffin pan. Bake, uncovered, in moderately slow oven about 20 minutes.
4 Meanwhile, make coffee syrup.
5 Stand cakes in pan 5 minutes, divide among plates; drizzle hot cakes with hot coffee syrup.

COFFEE SYRUP Stir sugar and the water in small saucepan over low heat until sugar dissolves; bring to a boil. Reduce heat; simmer, uncovered, without stirring, about 15 minutes or until syrup thickens. Stir in coffee; strain into small heatproof jug.

½ cup (50g) cocoa powder

1 cup (220g) firmly packed brown sugar

½ cup (125ml) boiling water

85g dark cooking chocolate, chopped finely

2 egg yolks

¼ cup (30g) almond meal

⅓ cup (50g) wholemeal plain flour

4 egg whites

COFFEE SYRUP
¾ cup (165g) firmly packed brown sugar

¾ cup (180ml) water

1 tablespoon instant coffee powder

NUTRITIONAL INFORMATION PER CAKE

5.1g total fat (2g saturated fat) **895kJ (214 cal)** 39.5g carbohydrate **4.2g protein** 1.2g fibre

rice pudding with raspberries

PREPARATION TIME 10 MINUTES **COOKING TIME** 1 HOUR 20 MINUTES **SERVES** 4

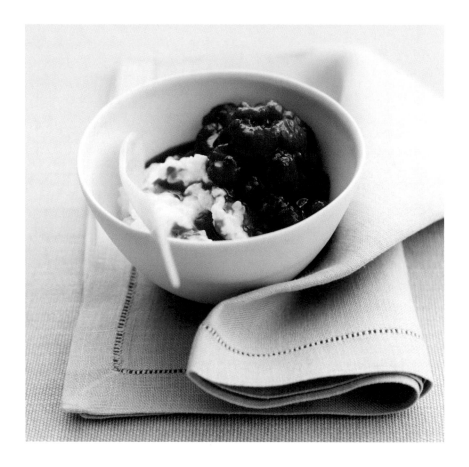

½ cup (100g) white short-grain rice

2 cups (500ml) milk

1 cup (250ml) skim milk

1 teaspoon vanilla extract

¼ cup (55g) caster sugar

RASPBERRY COMPOTE

300g frozen raspberries

1 tablespoon caster sugar

1 Preheat oven to moderately slow.
2 Rinse rice well under cold water; drain. Spread rice over bottom of shallow 1-litre (4-cup) baking dish.
3 Combine milks, extract and sugar in medium saucepan; bring to a boil. Pour hot milk mixture carefully over rice in baking dish; mix gently with fork. Cover dish tightly with foil; bake in moderately hot oven about 1 hour 15 minutes or until rice is softened and almost all liquid absorbed.
4 Meanwhile, combine raspberry compote ingredients in small saucepan; stir over low heat until sugar dissolves. Cool 10 minutes.
5 Serve compote with pudding.

NUTRITIONAL IN FORMATION PER SERVING

5.4g total fat (3.3g saturated fat) **1237kJ (296 cal)** 52.1g carbohydrate **9.6g protein** 4.3g fibre

pavlova roll with banana, kiwi and passionfruit

PREPARATION TIME 25 MINUTES **COOKING TIME** 20 MINUTES **SERVES** 10

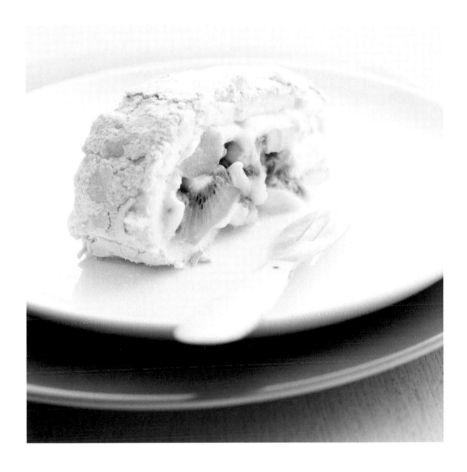

1 Preheat oven to moderately slow. Grease 25cm x 30cm swiss roll pan; line base with baking paper, extending paper 5cm over long sides of pan.

2 Beat egg whites in small bowl with electric mixer until soft peaks form. Gradually add caster sugar, 1 tablespoon at a time, beating until sugar dissolves between additions; fold in cornflour, vinegar and extract. Spread meringue mixture into prepared pan; bake, uncovered, in moderately slow oven about 20 minutes or until browned lightly.

3 Turn meringue onto sheet of baking paper sprinkled with half of the sifted icing sugar; remove lining paper, trim short ends of meringue.

4 Beat cream and remaining sifted icing sugar in small bowl with electric mixer until soft peaks form. Spread cream mixture over slightly warm meringue; place fruit lengthways along centre of meringue. Roll meringue firmly from long side, using paper as a guide. Refrigerate until ready to serve.

4 egg whites

¾ cup (165g) caster sugar

1 teaspoon cornflour

1 teaspoon white vinegar

1 teaspoon vanilla extract

1 tablespoon icing sugar mixture

300ml thickened light cream

1 large banana (230g), halved lengthways, sliced thinly

2 medium kiwifruit (170g), quartered lengthways

⅓ cup (80ml) passionfruit pulp, approximately four passionfruit

NUTRITIONAL INFORMATION PER SERVING

8.1g total fat (5.3g saturated fat) **748kJ (179 cal)** 24.6g carbohydrate **3g protein** 1.9g fibre

A peachy way to
end a perfect meal.

spiced stone-fruit strudel

PREPARATION TIME 20 MINUTES **COOKING TIME** 25 MINUTES **SERVES** 4

2 medium peaches (300g),
quartered, sliced thinly

2 medium nectarines (340g),
quartered, sliced thinly

2 tablespoons brown sugar

½ cup (80g) sultanas

1½ teaspoons ground cinnamon

½ teaspoon ground nutmeg

⅓ cup (25g) fresh breadcrumbs

6 sheets fillo pastry

20g butter, melted

2 tablespoons milk

2 teaspoons icing sugar mixture

1 Combine peach, nectarine, brown sugar, sultanas, spices and
breadcrumbs in medium bowl.
2 Preheat oven to moderately hot. Grease oven tray and line with
baking paper.
3 Stack fillo sheets, brushing all sheets lightly with half of the
combined butter and milk. Cut fillo stack in half widthways;
cover one stack with baking paper, then with a damp tea towel,
to prevent drying out.
4 Place half of the fruit mixture along centre of uncovered fillo stack;
roll from one side to enclose filling, sealing ends of roll with a little
of the remaining butter mixture. Place strudel, seam-side down, on
prepared tray; brush all over with a little of the remaining butter
mixture. Repeat process with remaining fillo stack, fruit mixture
and butter mixture.
5 Bake strudels, uncovered, in moderately hot oven about 25 minutes
or until browned lightly. Cut each strudel in half widthways; divide
among plates, dust with sifted icing sugar.

TIP You can use canned peaches and nectarines if fresh ones
aren't available.

NUTRITIONAL INFORMATION PER SERVING

5.5g total fat (3.1g saturated fat) **1191kJ (285 cal)** 53.1g carbohydrate **5.9g protein** 4.2g fibre

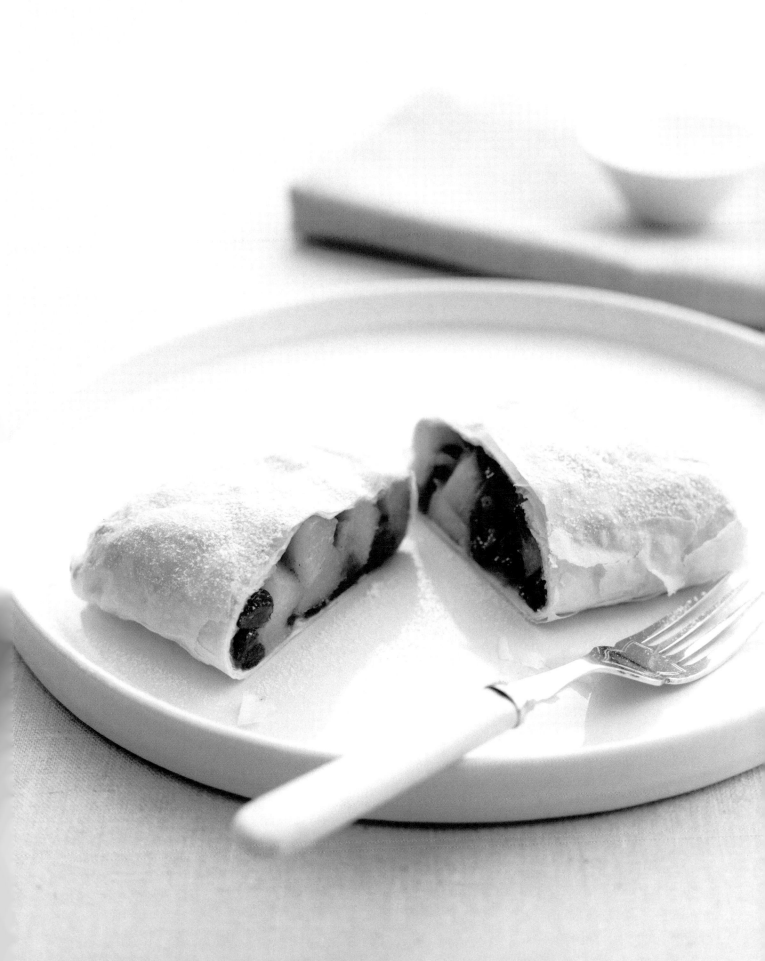

Old recipe, new trick
– layer biscuit, fruit
and cream cheese in
a tumbler to create
a charming parfait.

cherry cheesecake parfaits

PREPARATION TIME 15 MINUTES (PLUS REFRIGERATION TIME)
COOKING TIME 10 MINUTES **SERVES** 4

1 tablespoon caster sugar

1 tablespoon kirsch

425g can seeded black cherries, undrained

2 teaspoons cornflour

1 tablespoon water

60g low-fat cream cheese

200g low-fat french cheesecake yogurt

4 savoiardi sponge finger biscuits (50g), halved

1 Stir sugar, kirsch and cherries in small saucepan over low heat until sugar dissolves; bring to a boil. Remove from heat; reserve ⅔ cup cherry liquid from pan.
2 Return pan to heat, add blended cornflour and the water; cook, stirring, until cherry mixture boils and thickens slightly. Remove from heat; cool 10 minutes.
3 Meanwhile, beat cream cheese with yogurt in small bowl until combined.
4 Dip biscuit halves, one at a time, in reserved cherry liquid. Divide biscuit halves among four ¾-cup (180ml) glasses; top each with ⅓ cup of the cherry mixture then a quarter of the cream-cheese mixture. Refrigerate parfaits, covered, 30 minutes before serving.

NUTRITIONAL INFORMATION PER SERVING

4g total fat (2.4g saturated fat) **790kJ (189 cal)** 32.3g carbohydrate **5.3g protein** 1g fibre

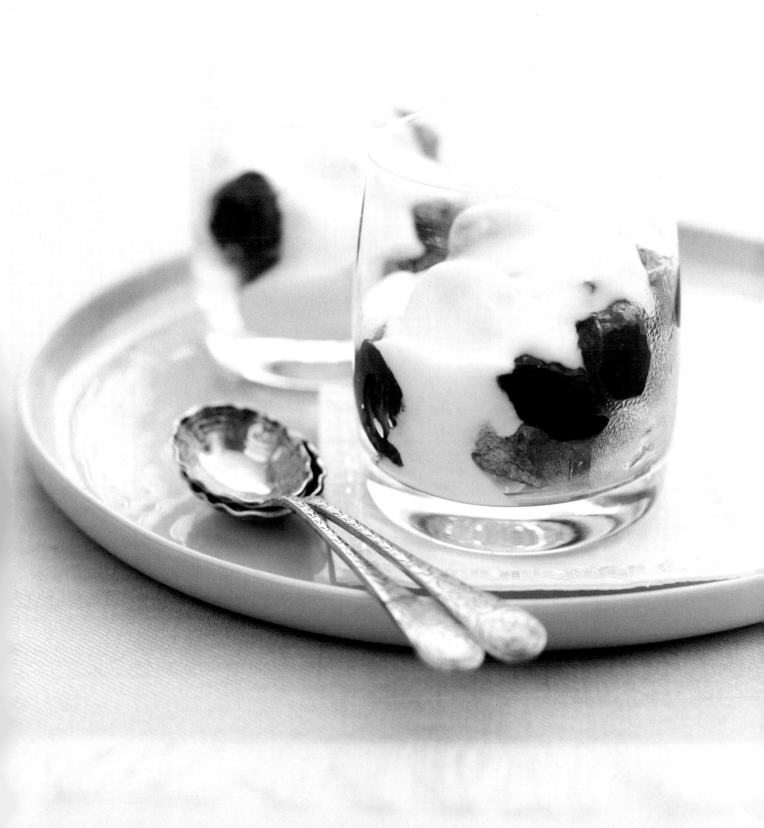

TREATS

Pamper your taste buds and comfort your soul with these mouth-watering morsels.

banana muffins with crunchy topping

PREPARATION TIME 20 MINUTES **COOKING TIME** 20 MINUTES **MAKES** 12

You need approximately two large (460g) overripe bananas for this recipe.

1¾ cups (280g) wholemeal self-raising flour

¾ cup (165g) firmly packed brown sugar

1 cup mashed banana

1 egg, beaten lightly

1 cup (250ml) buttermilk

¼ cup (60ml) vegetable oil

CRUNCHY OAT TOPPING

1 cup (90g) rolled oats

½ teaspoon ground nutmeg

2 tablespoons honey

1 Preheat oven to moderately hot. Lightly grease 12-hole (⅓-cup/80ml) muffin pan.

2 Make crunchy oat topping.

3 Sift flour and sugar into large bowl; stir in banana, egg, buttermilk and oil. Divide mixture among prepared holes of muffin pan; sprinkle with topping. Bake, uncovered, in moderately hot oven about 20 minutes. Stand muffins in pan 5 minutes; turn onto wire rack to cool.

CRUNCHY OAT TOPPING Blend or process oats until coarsely chopped. Combine oats, nutmeg and honey in small bowl.

NUTRITIONAL INFORMATION PER MUFFIN

6.6g total fat (1.2g saturated fat) **1041kJ (249 cal)** 42.5g carbohydrate **5.6g protein** 3.7g fibre

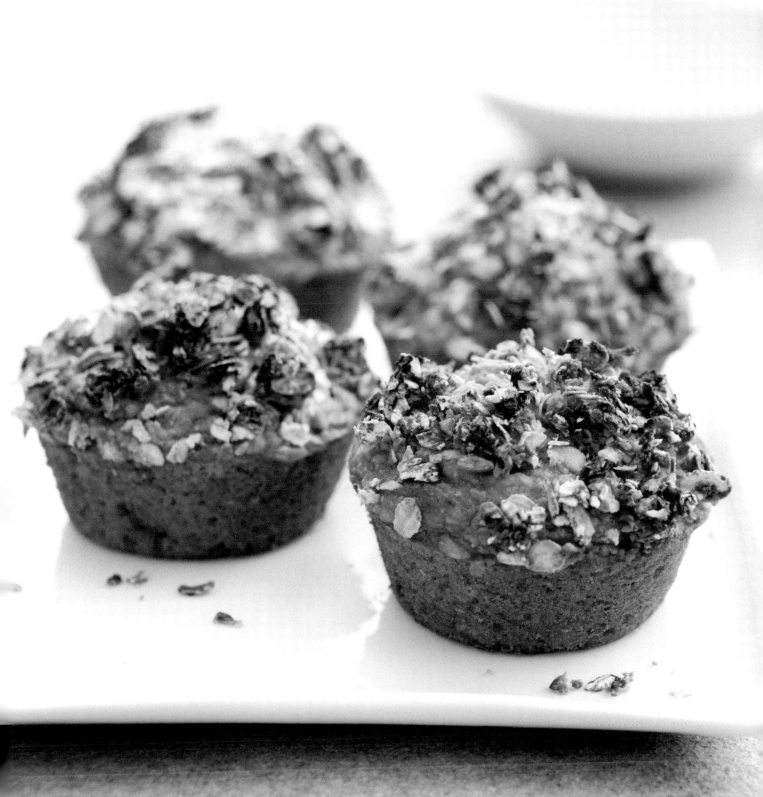

polenta and cottage cheese muffins

PREPARATION TIME 20 MINUTES **COOKING TIME** 20 MINUTES **MAKES** 12

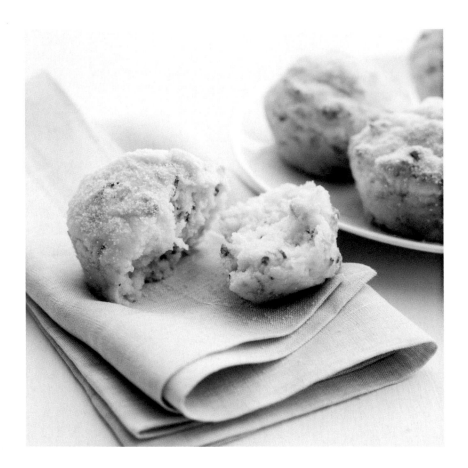

2 cups (300g) self-raising flour

2 teaspoons caster sugar

½ cup (85g) polenta

250g low-fat cottage cheese

⅓ cup (25g) coarsely grated parmesan cheese

½ teaspoon dried chilli flakes

4 green onions, chopped finely

1 egg

1 cup (250ml) skim milk

2 tablespoons vegetable oil

1 Preheat oven to moderately hot. Lightly grease 12-hole (⅓-cup/80ml) muffin pan.

2 Combine flour, sugar and ⅓ cup of the polenta in medium bowl with cottage cheese, parmesan, chilli and onion. Stir in combined egg, milk and oil. Divide mixture among prepared holes of muffin pan; sprinkle with remaining polenta. Bake, uncovered, in moderately hot oven about 20 minutes. Stand muffins in pan 5 minutes; turn onto wire rack to cool.

NUTRITIONAL INFORMATION PER MUFFIN

5.2g total fat (1.4g saturated fat) **796kJ (184 cal)** 25.8g carbohydrate **8.5g protein** 1.2g fibre

blueberry scones with vanilla frûche

PREPARATION TIME 10 MINUTES   **COOKING TIME** 20 MINUTES   **MAKES** 8

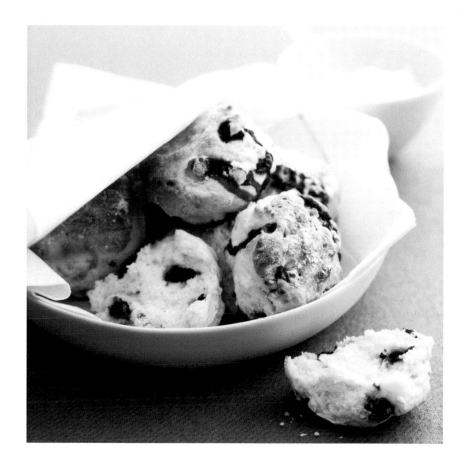

1 Preheat oven to hot. Grease shallow 20cm-round sandwich pan.
2 Sift flour and icing sugar into large bowl; pour in enough buttermilk to mix to a sticky dough. Fold in blueberries.
3 Gently knead dough on lightly floured surface until smooth; use hand to flatten out dough to about a 3cm thickness. Cut eight 5.5cm rounds from dough; place rounds, slightly touching, in prepared pan. Bake, uncovered, in hot oven about 20 minutes or until browned lightly; turn scones onto wire rack. Serve with Frûche.

2 cups (300g) self-raising flour
2 tablespoons icing sugar mixture
1¼ cups (310ml) buttermilk
150g blueberries
200g French Vanilla Frûche Lite

TIP To prevent dough from sticking, dust the inside of the cutter with flour.

NUTRITIONAL INFORMATION PER SCONE

2.6g total fat (1.5g saturated fat) **832kJ (199 cal)** 36.2g carbohydrate **7.1g protein** 1.8g fibre

chocolate rum and raisin loaf

PREPARATION TIME 30 MINUTES (PLUS STANDING TIME) **COOKING TIME** 45 MINUTES **SERVES** 12

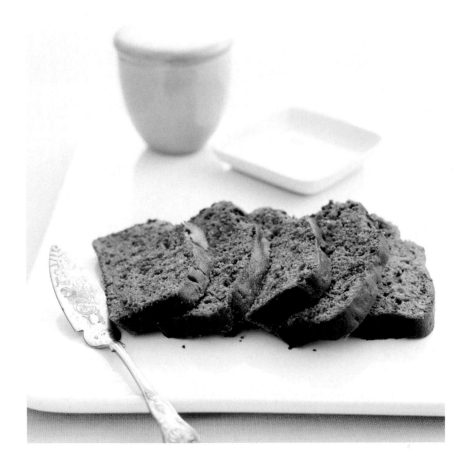

¾ cup (125g) raisins, chopped finely

¼ cup (60ml) dark rum

½ cup (110g) caster sugar

1 egg

1 teaspoon vanilla extract

2 tablespoons golden syrup

80g butter, melted

¾ cup (180ml) buttermilk

1 cup (150g) self-raising flour

2 tablespoons cocoa powder

¼ teaspoon ground nutmeg

⅓ cup (65g) dark Choc Bits, chopped coarsely

1 Preheat oven to moderate. Lightly grease 14cm x 21cm loaf pan; line base and two long sides with baking paper, extending paper 5cm above edges of pan.

2 Combine raisins and rum in small bowl; stand, covered, 2 hours.

3 Beat sugar, egg, extract and syrup in small bowl with electric mixer until thick and creamy.

4 Transfer mixture to medium bowl; stir in butter, buttermilk and sifted flour, cocoa and nutmeg. Stir in undrained raisin mixture and Choc Bits.

5 Spread mixture into prepared pan; bake, uncovered, in moderate oven about 45 minutes. Stand 10 minutes; turn onto wire rack to cool.

NUTRITIONAL INFORMATION PER SERVING

7.7g total fat (4.9g saturated fat) **932kJ (223 cal)** 33.6g carbohydrate **3.2g protein** 1.1g fibre

craisin, apricot and currant rock cakes

PREPARATION TIME 15 MINUTES **COOKING TIME** 15 MINUTES **MAKES** 20

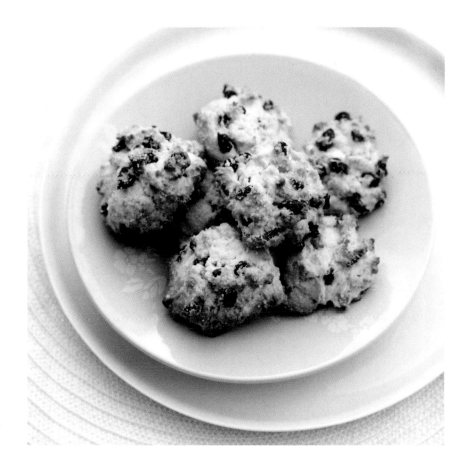

1 Preheat oven to moderately hot. Lightly grease two oven trays.
2 Combine flour and cinnamon in large bowl; rub in butter. Stir in caster sugar, fruit, egg and enough milk to give a moist but still firm consistency.
3 Drop rounded tablespoons of mixture about 5cm apart on prepared trays; sprinkle with raw sugar. Bake, uncovered, in moderately hot oven about 15 minutes or until browned lightly. Loosen cakes; cool on trays.

2 cups (300g) self-raising flour

¼ teaspoon ground cinnamon

90g cold butter, chopped

⅓ cup (75g) caster sugar

½ cup (75g) dried currants

½ cup (75g) dried apricots, chopped coarsely

½ cup (75g) craisins

1 egg, beaten lightly

½ cup (125ml) milk, approximately

1 tablespoon raw sugar

NUTRITIONAL INFORMATION PER CAKE

4.2g total fat (2.6g saturated fat) **564kJ (135 cal)** 22.4g carbohydrate **2.4g protein** 1.3g fibre

date and apple muesli slice

PREPARATION TIME 15 MINUTES **COOKING TIME** 35 MINUTES **MAKES** 32

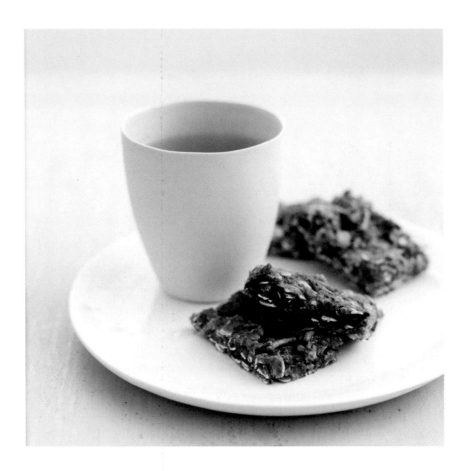

2 medium apples (300g), grated coarsely

2 tablespoons lemon juice

¼ cup (60ml) water

50g butter

2 cups (340g) seeded dates

2 cups (220g) natural muesli

1 cup (220g) firmly packed brown sugar

1 cup (150g) plain flour

1 teaspoon ground cinnamon

1 Preheat oven to moderate. Lightly grease 25cm x 30cm swiss roll pan.
2 Combine apple, juice, the water, butter and dates in medium saucepan; bring to a boil. Reduce heat; simmer, covered, about 5 minutes or until apple is soft. Uncover; cook, stirring occasionally, about 5 minutes or until mixture thickens to a paste-like consistency.
3 Meanwhile, place muesli in large frying pan; stir over low heat about 5 minutes or until browned lightly. Combine muesli in large bowl with sugar, flour and cinnamon. Stir in date mixture.
4 Spread slice mixture into prepared pan; bake, uncovered, in moderate oven about 20 minutes or until firm. Cool in pan before cutting.

NUTRITIONAL INFORMATION PER SLICE

1.6g total fat (1g saturated fat) **326kJ (79 cal)** 15.6g carbohydrate **1g protein** 1g fibre

spicy parmesan seed twists

PREPARATION TIME 15 MINUTES **COOKING TIME** 15 MINUTES **MAKES** 24

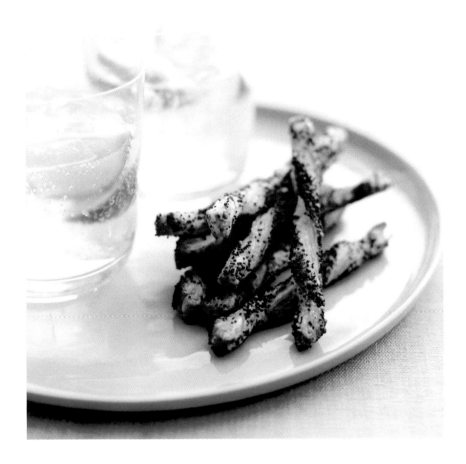

1 Preheat oven to moderately hot. Grease and line two oven trays.
2 Brush pastry halves with egg on one side; sprinkle with combined seeds, paprika and salt. Turn over one of the halves so unseeded side faces up; brush with egg, sprinkle with parmesan. Sandwich the two halves with parmesan side in the centre and two seeded sides facing out; press down firmly.
3 Cut pastry widthways into 24 strips; twist each strip, pinching ends to seal. Place twists on prepared trays; bake, uncovered, in moderately hot oven about 15 minutes or until browned lightly.

1 sheet ready-rolled
puff pastry, halved

1 egg yolk

1 tablespoon poppy seeds

2 teaspoons mustard seeds

1 teaspoon sweet paprika

½ teaspoon salt

2 tablespoons finely grated
parmesan cheese

NUTRITIONAL INFORMATION PER TWIST

2.2g total fat (1.1g saturated fat) **138kJ (33 cal)** 2.5g carbohydrate **0.8g protein** 0.2g fibre

almond macaroons

PREPARATION TIME 30 MINUTES **COOKING TIME** 10 MINUTES **MAKES** 28

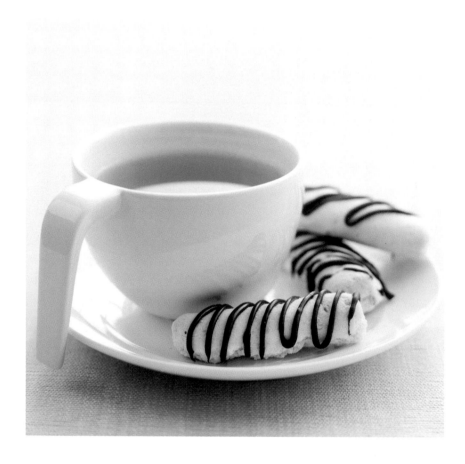

1 egg white

⅔ cup (150g) caster sugar

¼ teaspoon almond extract

1 cup (125g) almond meal

½ cup (70g) toasted slivered almonds, chopped coarsely

50g dark chocolate Melts, melted

1 Preheat oven to moderate. Lightly grease and line two oven trays.

2 Beat egg white in small bowl with electric mixer until soft peaks form. Gradually add sugar, 1 tablespoon at a time, beating until sugar dissolves between additions. Transfer egg-white mixture to medium bowl; fold in extract, almond meal and nuts.

3 Divide mixture in half; roll each half into 20cm log. Cut each log into 14 pieces; roll each piece into 6cm log. Place logs on prepared trays; bake, uncovered, in moderate oven about 8 minutes. Cool on trays; drizzle or pipe macaroons with melted chocolate.

NUTRITIONAL INFORMATION PER MACAROON

4.3g total fat (0.6g saturated fat) **297kJ (71 cal)** 6.8g carbohydrate **1.6g protein** 0.6g fibre

orange toffee popcorn

PREPARATION TIME 5 MINUTES **COOKING TIME** 30 MINUTES **SERVES** 4

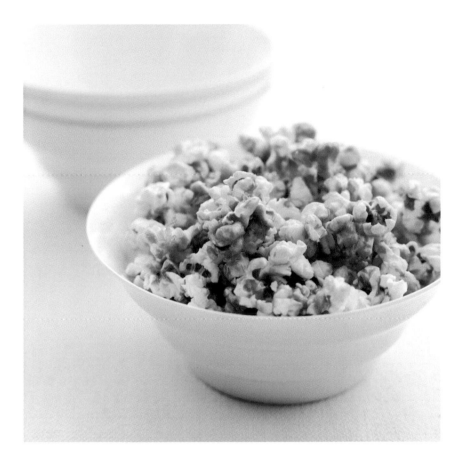

1 Combine sugar with the water in medium heavy-based saucepan. Stir over low heat, without boiling, until sugar dissolves; bring to a boil. Reduce heat; simmer, uncovered, without stirring, about 25 minutes or until toffee is golden brown in colour.

2 Meanwhile, heat oil in large saucepan. Add corn, cover with tight-fitting lid; cook about 5 minutes, shaking pan occasionally, until popping stops. Lightly grease large baking dish; spread popcorn evenly in dish, sprinkle with rind.

3 Working quickly, drizzle toffee over popcorn; using metal spatula, toss to combine, cool 5 minutes. Break popcorn into bowls to serve.

1½ cups (330g) caster sugar

1½ cups (375ml) water

1 tablespoon vegetable oil

½ cup (115g) popping corn

1 tablespoon coarsely grated orange rind

NUTRITIONAL INFORMATION PER SERVING

5.8g total fat (0.8g saturated fat) **1864kJ (446 cal)** 98.6g carbohydrate **3.4g protein** 6.4g fibre

glossary

ALL-BRAN a low-fat, high-fibre bran-based breakfast cereal.

ALLSPICE also known as pimento or jamaican pepper; so-named because is tastes like a combination of nutmeg, cumin, clove and cinnamon – all spices.

ALMONDS
essence often interchangeable with extract; made with almond oil and alcohol or another agent.
flaked paper-thin slices.
meal also known as ground almonds; nuts are powdered to a coarse flour texture.
slivered cut lengthways.

BEAN SPROUTS also known as bean shoots; tender new growths of beans and seeds especially germinated for consumption as sprouts.

BEANS
borlotti also known as roman beans.
green also known as french or string beans.

BEETROOT also known as red beets; firm, round root vegetable.

BOK CHOY also known as bak choy, pak choi, chinese white cabbage or chinese chard; has a fresh, mild mustard taste. Use both stems and leaves.
baby bok choy also known as pak kat farang or shanghai bok choy; is small and more tender than bok choy.

BRIOCHE rich, French yeast-risen bread made with butter and eggs. Available from pâtisseries or specialty bread shops.

BUTTERMILK sold in the dairy compartments in supermarkets. Low in fat and is a good substitution for dairy products such as cream or sour cream.

CAPSICUM also known as bell pepper or, simply, pepper. Native to Central and South America. Discard seeds and membranes before use.

CAYENNE PEPPER long, thin-fleshed, extremely hot, dried red chilli, usually purchased ground; both arbol and guajillo chillies are the fresh sources for cayenne.

CHEESE
fetta a crumbly goat- or sheep-milk cheese with a sharp salty taste.
goat made from goats milk, has a strong, earthy taste; available in both soft and firm textures, sometimes rolled in ash or herbs.
light cream the light version of Philadelphia Cream Cheese. Is a blend of cottage and cream cheeses with a fat content of 21%.

CHICKPEAS also called channa, garbanzos or hummus; a sandy-coloured, irregularly round legume used extensively in Latin and Mediterranean cooking.

CHILLI Use rubber gloves when seeding and chopping fresh chillies as they can burn your skin. Removing seeds and membranes lessens the heat level.
flakes crushed dried chillies.
green generally unripened thai chillies, but different varieties that are ripe when green may be used, such as habanero, poblano or serrano chillies.
thai, red small, medium hot, and bright red in colour.

CHINESE CABBAGE also known as peking or napa cabbage, wong bok or petsai; elongated in shape with pale green, crinkly leaves.

CHOC BITS also known as chocolate chips and chocolate morsels; available in milk, white and dark chocolate.

CHOCOLATE MELTS discs of compounded chocolate ideal for melting or moulding.

CIABATTA in Italian, the word means slipper, which is the traditional shape of this crisp-crusted white bread.

COCOA POWDER also known as cocoa; dried, unsweetened, roasted and ground cocoa beans.

COCONUT
cream is obtained commercially from the first pressing of the coconut flesh alone, without the addition of water.
shredded thin strips of dried coconut.

COOKING-OIL SPRAY we used a cholesterol-free cooking spray made from canola oil.

CORNFLOUR also known as cornstarch; used as a thickening agent in all types of cooking.

CORNICHON French for gherkin, a tiny variety of cucumber. Pickled, they are a traditional accompaniment to pâté.

COUSCOUS a fine, grain-like cereal product, made from semolina. Originally from North Africa.

CRAISINS dried cranberries.

CUMIN also known as zeera, available in seed or ground form.

DASHI basic seaweed and fish stock. Made from dried bonito (fish) flakes and kelp (kombu). Instant dashi powder, also known as dashi-no-moto, is a concentrated granulated powder. Available from Asian specialty stores.

EGGPLANT also known as aubergine; ranges in size from tiny to very large and in colour from pale green to deep purple.

FENNEL also known as finocchio or anise; eaten raw in salads or braised or fried as a vegetable accompaniment. Also the name given to dried seeds having a licorice flavour.

FLOUR
plain an all-purpose flour, made from wheat.
self-raising plain flour sifted with baking powder (1 cup flour to 2 teaspoons baking powder).

FOCACCIA a flat Italian-style bread.

FRUCHE commercial dessert with less than 0.5g fat per 100g. Similar to fromage frais.

GELATINE we used powdered gelatine; also available in sheet form known as leaf gelatine.

GINGER
fresh also known as green or root ginger. Can be kept, peeled, covered with dry sherry, in a jar and refrigerated, or frozen in an airtight container.
ground also known as powdered ginger; cannot be substituted for fresh ginger.
pickled available, packaged, from Asian food stores; pickled paper-thin shavings of ginger in a mixture of vinegar, sugar and natural colouring.

GRAPEVINE LEAVES available fresh or Cryovac-packed in brine. Available from Middle-Eastern food stores.

GREEN SPLIT PEAS also known as field peas; green or yellow pulse grown especially for drying, split in half along a centre seam.

HARISSA sauce or paste made from dried red chillies, garlic, oil and sometimes caraway seeds.

HERBS when specified, we used dried (not ground) herbs in the proportion of 1:4 for fresh herbs (1 teaspoon dried herbs equals 4 teaspoons chopped fresh herbs).

coriander also known as cilantro or chinese parsley. Also sold as seeds, whole or ground.

parsley, flat-leaf also known as continental or italian parsley.

thai basil has smaller leaves and purplish stems. It has a slight licorice or aniseed taste, and is often used in Thai cuisine.

HORSERADISH CREAM a paste made of grated horseradish, oil, mustard seeds and sugar.

HUMMUS a Middle Eastern dip or salad made from chickpeas, garlic, lemon juice and tahini (sesame seed paste).

KAFFIR LIME LEAVES look like two glossy dark green leaves joined end to end, forming a rounded hourglass shape. Sold fresh, dried or frozen; the dried leaves are less potent so double the number called for in a recipe if you substitute them for fresh leaves. A strip of fresh lime peel may be substituted for each kaffir lime leaf.

KIRSCH cherry-flavoured liqueur.

KUMARA orange-fleshed sweet potato often confused with yam.

LAMINGTON PAN 20cm x 30cm slab cake pan, 3cm deep.

LEBANESE CUCUMBER short, slender and thin-skinned; this variety is also known as the burpless or european cucumber.

LEMON GRASS a tall, clumping, lemon-smelling and tasting, sharp-edged grass; the white lower part of the stem is used, finely chopped, in cooking.

MIRIN a champagne-coloured Japanese cooking wine made expressly for cooking and should not be confused with sake.

MIXED SPICE a blend of ground spices usually consisting of cinnamon, allspice and nutmeg.

MUSHROOMS
flat large, flat mushrooms with a rich earthy flavour; sometimes misnamed field mushrooms, which are wild mushrooms.

oyster also known as abalone; grey-white mushroom shaped like a fan.

shiitake when fresh are also known as chinese black, forest or golden oak mushrooms. Are large and meaty with an earthy taste of wild mushrooms. When dried, they are known as donko or dried chinese mushrooms; rehydrate before use.

swiss brown also known as roman or cremini; light-to dark-brown mushrooms with full-bodied flavour. Button or cap mushrooms can be substituted.

NASHI also called japanese or asian pear; a member of the pear family, but similar in appearance to an apple.

NORI a type of dried seaweed often used in Japanese cooking. Sold in thin sheets.

NUTMEG available whole or in ground form.

PINE NUTS a small, cream-coloured kernel from pine cones; known as pignoli.

PITTA also known as lebanese bread. Is also available in small thick pieces called pocket pitta.

POLENTA also known as cornmeal; a flour-like cereal made of dried corn (maize), also the name of the dish made from it.

PRESERVED LEMON whole or quartered salted lemons preserved in a mixture of olive oil and lemon juice; imparts a rich, salty-sour acidic flavour. Available from good food shops and delicatessens. Rinse well under cold water before using.

PROSCIUTTO cured, air-dried (unsmoked), pressed ham.

RAISINS dried, sweet grapes.

RICE
arborio small, round-grain rice able to absorb large amounts of liquid; suitable for risottos.

koshihikari small, round-grain white rice. May be substituted with short-grain white rice.

ROLLED RICE flattened rice grain rolled into flakes; appearance is similar to rolled oats.

SAKE Japanese rice wine. If unavailable, dry sherry, vermouth or brandy may be substituted.

SAMBAL OELEK also spelled ulek or olek; a salty paste made from ground chillies and vinegar.

SAUCES
cranberry made of cranberries cooked in sugar syrup; has an astringent flavour.

kecap manis a dark, thick, sweet soy sauce used in most South-East Asian cuisines.

SAVOIARDI SPONGE FINGER BISCUITS also known as savoy biscuits, lady's fingers or sponge fingers; Italian-style crisp fingers made from sponge cake mixture.

SHALLOTS also called french shallots, golden shallots or eschalots; small, elongated, brown-skinned members of the onion family.

SICHUAN PEPPERCORNS also known as szechuan or chinese pepper. Small, red-brown aromatic seeds with a distinctive mild peppery-lemon flavour.

SOBA thin spaghetti-like pale brown noodle from Japan made from varying amounts of buckwheat and wheat flour. Used in soups and stir-fries.

STAR ANISE a star-shaped pod whose seeds have an astringent aniseed flavour; used to flavour stocks.

SUGAR
brown a soft, fine granulated sugar retaining molasses for its characteristic colour and flavour.

caster also known as superfine or finely granulated table sugar.

icing sugar mixture also known as confectioners' sugar or powdered sugar.

palm also known as nam tan pip, jaggery or gula melaka. Sold in rock-hard cakes; can be substituted with brown sugar.

raw natural brown granulated sugar.

SUMAC a purple-red, astringent spice that adds a tart, lemony flavour. Found in Middle-Eastern food stores.

TORTILLA unleavened bread originating in Mexico; made from either wheat or corn.

TURMERIC also known as kamin; known for the golden colour it imparts to dishes.

TZATZIKI Greek yogurt and cucumber dish sometimes containing mint and/or garlic.

index

almond macaroons 114
apple and date
   muesli slice 112
apple oaty pikelets 10
apricot, craisin and
   currant rock cakes 111
bacon with maple-
   syrup flavoured
   borlotti beans 16
balsamic-seared steak
   with kipflers and
   mushrooms 73
banana and caramel
   sauce with brown-
   sugar meringues 90
banana muffins with
   crunchy topping 106
barley risotto with chicken
   and tarragon 26
beans, borlotti, maple-
   syrup flavoured,
   with bacon 16
beef fillet with vegetable
   and polenta chips,
   pepper-crusted 86
beef, roast, and
   horseradish cream
   on focaccia 22
beetroot risotto
   with rocket 41
beetroot, lentil and
   rocket salad 19
berry compote, soufflé 6
berry stack, summer 95
bircher muesli, peach 12
blueberry scones with
   vanilla frûche 109
blue-eye kebabs with
   almond and lemon
   couscous, moroccan 52
bruschetta
   with smoked salmon,
      cream cheese and
      rocket 15
   with strawberry, banana
      and ricotta 14
   with ham, tomato
      and avocado 24
   with prawn and lime
      mayonnaise 24
   with smoked chicken
      and mango chutney 25
   with tuna salad 25
cakes, chocolate fudge
   with coffee syrup 99
cakes, rock, craisin,
   apricot and currant 111
cheesecake parfaits,
   cherry 104
chicken
   and corn soup 20
   and peach salad 18
   and tarragon with
      barley risotto 26

caramelised onion
   and fig pizza 37
donburi 89
herb-stuffed, with
   tomato salad 69
honey dijon, with
   creamy celery and
   fennel slaw 55
noodle soup, thai 21
salad, shredded 48
smoked, and mango
   chutney bruschetta 25
tortilla roll with sprout
   and herb salad 78
chickpea salad 18
chocolate fudge cakes
   with coffee syrup 99
chocolate rum and
   raisin loaf 110
corn and chicken soup 20
craisin, apricot and
   currant rock cakes 111
curry lamb and lentil 81
date and apple
   muesli slice 112
donburi, chicken 89
eggplant, lamb and
   grapevine leaves,
   layered 29
eggs ranchero-style 17
eggs, poached,
   on sourdough 9
figs, caramelised,
   with spiced yogurt 93
fish with sumac, salt
   and pepper and
   mediterranean salad 74
french onion soup 21
ginger muffins with stewed
   pear, day before 11
gnocchi, kumara, with
   rocket and basil pesto 30
honey dijon chicken
   with creamy celery
   and fennel slaw 55
kiwi fruit sorbet 96
koshari 60
kumara gnocchi with rocket
   and basil pesto 30
lamb and barley salad,
   chilli coriander 33
lamb and lentil curry 81
lamb cutlets, grilled, with
   warm risoni salad 82
lamb, eggplant and
   grapevine leaves,
   layered 29
lamb, harissa-scented,
   with char-grilled
   vegetables 85
lamb, tabbouleh and
   hummus on pitta 22
lentil, rocket and
   beetroot salad 19

mango sorbet 96
meringues, brown-sugar,
   with banana and
   caramel sauce 90
muesli slice,
   date and apple 112
muesli, peach bircher 12
muffins with crunchy
   topping, banana 106
muffins, ginger with
   stewed pear 11
muffins, polenta and
   cottage cheese 108
mushrooms, sautéed,
   on toast 8
mussels, thai-flavoured 70
oaty apple pikelets 10
onion soup, french 21
orange toffee popcorn 115
pappardelle with roasted
   tomato, spinach
   and ricotta 38
parmesan seed
   twists, spicy 113
passionfruit yogurt,
   frozen 92
pavlova roll with banana,
   kiwi and passionfruit 101
pea and mint puree
   with prawn ravioli 59
pea, ricotta, mint and
   spinach sandwich 23
peach bircher muesli 12
pepper-crusted beef fillet
   with vegetable and
   polenta chips 86
pikelets, oaty apple 10
pineapple sorbet 96
pizza, chicken, fig and
   caramelised onion 37
polenta and cottage
   cheese muffins 108
popcorn, orange toffee 115
pork cutlets with spinach
   and pecan salad,
   orange-glazed 34
pork salad with kaffir
   lime dressing, thai 47
porridge with dried
   fruit compote 13
prawn ravioli with mint
   and pea puree 59
pumpkin and
   split pea tagine 42
raspberries with
   rice pudding 100
ravioli, prawn, with mint
   and pea puree 59
rice pudding with
   raspberries 100
risotto, barley, with
   chicken and tarragon 26
risotto, beetroot,
   with rocket 41

salmon, asian-spiced,
   with nashi, mint and
   coriander salad 51
sandwich, pea, ricotta,
   mint and spinach 23
scones, blueberry,
   with vanilla frûche 109
snapper, grilled, with
   spicy tomato sauce 62
soba, chilled, with
   seared tuna 77
sorbet,
   kiwi fruit 96
   mango 96
   pineapple 96
sorbets, tropical fruit 96
soufflé with
   berry compote 6
soup
   chicken and corn 20
   french onion 21
   risoni and spring
      vegetable 20
   thai chicken noodle 21
spicy parmesan
   seed twists 113
squid stuffed with smoked
   trout and basil 67
steak, balsamic-seared,
   with kipflers and
   mushrooms 73
strudel, spiced
   stone-fruit 102
tabbouleh, lamb and
   hummus on pitta 22
thai chicken
   noodle soup 21
thai-flavoured mussels 70
tortilla, glazed-chicken
   with sprout and
   herb salad 78
tropical fruit sorbets 96
trout in baby bok choy
   parcels, ocean 56
trout, smoked, and basil,
   squid stuffed with 67
trout, smoked, salad roll 23
tuna salad 19
tuna, seared, with
   chilled soba 77
veal cutlets with
   onion marmalade 65
veal, mushroom and
   fennel rolls with
   horseradish mash 44
vegetable, spring,
   and risoni soup 20
vegetables, char-grilled
   with harissa-scented
   lamb 85
yogurt, frozen
   passionfruit 92
yogurt, spiced, with
   caramelised figs 93

facts + figures

Wherever you live, you'll be able to use our recipes with the help of these easy-to-follow conversions. While these conversions are approximate only, the difference between an exact and the approximate conversion of various liquid and dry measures is minimal and will not affect your cooking results.

LIQUID MEASURES

METRIC	IMPERIAL
30ml	1 fluid oz
60ml	2 fluid oz
100ml	3 fluid oz
125ml	4 fluid oz
150ml	5 fluid oz (¼ pint/1 gill)
190ml	6 fluid oz
250ml	8 fluid oz
300ml	10 fluid oz (½ pint)
500ml	16 fluid oz
600ml	20 fluid oz (1 pint)
1000ml (1 litre)	1¾ pints

MEASURING EQUIPMENT

The difference between one country's measuring cups and another's is, at most, within a 2 or 3 teaspoon variance. (For the record, one Australian metric measuring cup holds approximately 250ml.) The most accurate way of measuring dry ingredients is to weigh them. When measuring liquids, use a clear glass or plastic jug with the metric markings. (One Australian metric tablespoon holds 20ml; one Australian metric teaspoon holds 5ml.)

DRY MEASURES

METRIC	IMPERIAL
15g	½oz
30g	1oz
60g	2oz
90g	3oz
125g	4oz (¼lb)
155g	5oz
185g	6oz
220g	7oz
250g	8oz (½lb)
280g	9oz
315g	10oz
345g	11oz
375g	12oz (¾lb)
410g	13oz
440g	14oz
470g	15oz
500g	16oz (1lb)
750g	24oz (1½lb)
1kg	32oz (2lb)

HELPFUL MEASURES

METRIC	IMPERIAL
3mm	⅛in
6mm	¼in
1cm	½in
2cm	¾in
2.5cm	1in
5cm	2in
6cm	2½in
8cm	3in
10cm	4in
13cm	5in
15cm	6in
18cm	7in
20cm	8in
23cm	9in
25cm	10in
28cm	11in
30cm	12in (1ft)

HOW TO MEASURE

When using graduated metric measuring cups, shake dry ingredients loosely into the appropriate cup. Do not tap the cup on a bench or tightly pack the ingredients unless directed to do so. Level top of measuring cups and measuring spoons with a knife. When measuring liquids, place a clear glass or plastic jug with metric markings on a flat surface to check accuracy at eye level.

Note: North America, NZ and the UK use 15ml tablespoons. All cup and spoon measurements are level.

We use large eggs having an average weight of 60g.

OVEN TEMPERATURES

These oven temperatures are only a guide. Always check the manufacturer's manual.

	°C (CELSIUS)	°F (FAHRENHEIT)	GAS MARK
Very slow	120	250	½
Slow	140-150	275-300	1-2
Moderately slow	170	325	3
Moderate	180-190	350-375	4-5
Moderately hot	200	400	6
Hot	220-230	425-450	7-8
Very hot	240	475	9

ARE YOU MISSING SOME OF THE WORLD'S FAVOURITE COOKBOOKS?

The Australian Women's Weekly Cookbooks are available from bookshops, cookshops, supermarkets and other stores all over the world. You can also buy direct from the publisher, using the order form below.

TITLE	RRP	QTY	TITLE	RRP	QTY
Almost Vegetarian	£5.99		French Food, New	£5.99	
Asian, Meals in Minutes	£5.99		Get Real, Make a Meal	£5.99	
Babies & Toddlers Good Food	£5.99		Good Food Fast	£5.99	
Barbecue Meals In Minutes	£5.99		Great Beef Cookbook	£5.99	
Basic Cooking Class	£5.99		Great Chicken Cookbook	£5.99	
Beginners Cooking Class	£5.99		Great Lamb Cookbook	£5.99	
Beginners Simple Meals	£5.99		Greek Cooking Class	£5.99	
Beginners Thai	£5.99		Healthy Heart Cookbook	£5.99	
Best Ever Slimmers' Recipes	£5.99		Indian Cooking Class	£5.99	
Best Food	£5.99		Italian Cooking Class	£5.99	
Best Food Desserts	£5.99		Japanese Cooking Class	£5.99	
Best Food Mains	£5.99		Kids' Birthday Cakes	£5.99	
Big Book of Beautiful Biscuits	£5.99		Kids Cooking	£5.99	
Biscuits & Slices	£5.99		Lean Food	£5.99	
Cakes & Slices Cookbook	£5.99		Low-fat Feasts	£5.99	
Cakes Cooking Class	£5.99		Low-fat Food For Life	£5.99	
Caribbean Cooking	£5.99		Low-fat Meals in Minutes	£5.99	
Casseroles	£5.99		Main Course Salads	£5.99	
Celebration Cakes	£5.99		Meals in Minutes	£5.99	
Chicken Meals in Minutes	£5.99		Mediterranean Cookbook	£5.99	
Chinese Cooking Class	£5.99		Middle Eastern Cooking Class	£5.99	
Christmas Book	£5.99		Midweek Meals in Minutes	£5.99	
Christmas Cooking	£5.99		Muffins, Scones & Bread	£5.99	
Cocktails	£5.99		New Finger Food	£5.99	
Cooking for Crowds	£5.99		Pasta Cookbook	£5.99	
Cooking for Friends	£5.99		Pasta Meals in Minutes	£5.99	
Cooking For Two	£5.99		Potatoes	£5.99	
Creative Cooking on a Budget	£5.99		Quick Meals in Minutes	£5.99	
Detox (Sept 05)	£5.99		Quick-mix Biscuits & Slices	£5.99	
Dinner Beef	£5.99		Quick-mix Cakes	£5.99	
Dinner Lamb (Aug 05)	£5.99		Salads: Simple, Fast & Fresh	£5.99	
Dinner Seafood	£5.99		Saucery	£5.99	
Easy Australian Style	£5.99		Sensational Stir-Fries	£5.99	
Easy Curry	£5.99		Short-order Cook	£5.99	
Easy Spanish-Style	£5.99		Sweet Old Fashioned Favourites	£5.99	
Easy Vietnamese-Style	£5.99		Thai Cooking Class	£5.99	
Essential Barbecue	£5.99		Vegetarian Meals in Minutes	£5.99	
Essential Microwave	£5.99		Weekend Cook	£5.99	
Essential Soup	£5.99		Wicked Sweet Indulgences	£5.99	
Freezer, Meals from the	£5.99		Wok, Meals in Minutes	£5.99	
French Cooking Class	£5.99		**TOTAL COST:**	**£**	

NAME _____

ADDRESS _____

_____ POSTCODE _____

DAYTIME PHONE _____

I ENCLOSE MY CHEQUE/MONEY ORDER FOR £ _____

OR PLEASE CHARGE MY VISA, ACCESS OR MASTERCARD NUMBER

_____

CARD HOLDER'S NAME _____

EXPIRY DATE _____

CARDHOLDER'S SIGNATURE _____

To order: Mail or fax — photocopy or complete the order form above, and send your credit card details or cheque payable to: Australian Consolidated Press (UK), Moulton Park Business Centre, Red House Road, Moulton Park, Northampton NN3 6AQ, phone (+44) (0) 1604 497531, fax (+44) (0) 1604 497533, e-mail books@acpuk.com

Non-UK residents: We accept the credit cards listed on the coupon, or cheques, drafts or International Money Orders payable in sterling and drawn on a UK bank. Credit card charges are at the exchange rate current at the time of payment.

Postage and packing: Within the UK, add £1.50 for one book or £3.00 for two books. There is no postal charge for orders of three or more books for delivery within the UK. For delivery outside the UK, please phone, fax or e-mail for a quote.

Offer ends 31.12.2005

Test Kitchen
Food director *Pamela Clark*
Food editor *Karen Hammial*
Assistant food editor *Amira Georgy*
Test Kitchen manager *Cathie Lonnie*
Home economists *Sammie Coryton,*
Nancy Duran, Elizabeth Macri,
Christina Martignago, Sharon Reeve,
Susie Riggall, Kirrily Smith
Editorial coordinator *Rebecca Steyns*
Nutritional information *Laila Ibram*

ACP Books
Editorial director *Susan Tomnay*
Creative director *Hieu Chi Nguyen*
Senior editors *Lynda Wilton, Wendy Bryant*
Contributing writer *Klay Lamprell*
Designer *Hieu Chi Nguyen*
Design assistant *Karen Lai*
Studio manager *Caryl Wiggins*
Editorial coordinator *Merryn Pearse*
Sales director *Brian Cearnes*
Publishing manager (rights & new projects)
 Jane Hazell
Marketing director *Nicole Pizanis*
Sales and marketing coordinator *Caroline Lowry*
Pre-press *Harry Palmer*
Production manager *Carol Currie*
Business manager *Seymour Cohen*
Business analyst *Martin Howes*
Chief executive officer *John Alexander*
Group publisher *Pat Ingram*
Publisher *Sue Wannan*
Editor-in-chief *Deborah Thomas*

Produced by ACP Books, Sydney.
Printed by Times Printers, Singapore.
Published by ACP Publishing Pty Limited,
54 Park St, Sydney; GPO Box 4088,
Sydney, NSW 2001.
Ph: (02) 9282 8618 Fax: (02) 9267 9438.
acpbooks@acp.com.au
www.acpbooks.com.au
To order books, phone 136 116.
Send recipe enquiries to:
recipeenquiries@acp.com.au
AUSTRALIA: Distributed by Network Services,
GPO Box 4088, Sydney, NSW 2001.
Ph: (02) 9282 8777 Fax: (02) 9264 3278.
UNITED KINGDOM: Distributed by Australian
Consolidated Press (UK), Moulton Park
Business Centre, Red House Rd,
Moulton Park, Northampton, NN3 6AQ.
Ph: (01604) 497531 Fax: (01604) 497533
acpukltd@aol.com
CANADA: Distributed by Whitecap Books Ltd,
351 Lynn Ave, North Vancouver, BC, V7J 2C4.
Ph: (604) 980 9852 Fax: (604) 980 8197
customerservice@whitecap.ca
www.whitecap.ca
NEW ZEALAND: Distributed by Netlink
Distribution Company, ACP Media Centre,
Cnr Fanshawe and Beaumont Streets,
Westhaven, Auckland.
PO Box 47906, Ponsonby, Auckland, NZ.
Ph: (09) 366 9966 ask@ndcnz.co.nz
SOUTH AFRICA: Distributed by PSD
Promotions, 30 Diesel Road Isando,
Gauteng Johannesburg.
PO Box 1175, Isando 1600,
Gauteng Johannesburg.
Ph: (2711) 392 6065 Fax: (2711) 392 6079
orders@psdprom.co.za

Clark, Pamela.
The Australian Women's Weekly
Slim: an eating plan for life.
Includes index.
ISBN 1 86396 403 7
1. Low-fat diet – recipes. I. Title.
II. Title: Slim: an eating plan for life.
III. Title: Australian Women's Weekly.

641.56384
© ACP Publishing Pty Limited 2004
ABN 18 053 273 546